Advance Praise for

The Body-Mind-Soul Solution: Healing Emotional Pain through Exercise

"This is a groundbreaking book with a most unique and satisfying approach to healing emotional pain through exercise. I highly recommend this program to everybody who needs a fresh way to handle life's traumas and challenges."

—ANN LOUISE GITTLEMAN, PH.D., C.N.S.
Author of the *New York Times* bestsellers *The Fat Flush Plan*
and *Before the Change*

"Livingstone uniquely combines the positive aspect of physical exercise and self-help techniques as a way of dealing with our emotional pain. The book is user friendly and has many studies that help clarify his thoughts. This book can benefit anyone who exercises or is considering an exercise program."

—GERALD G. JAMPOLSKY, M.D.
Author of the *New York Times* bestseller *Love is Letting Go of Fear*

"I believe strongly in the concepts in this book. Exercise has been extremely therapeutic for me. Bob creates a productive and unique methodology in an easy to read fashion."

—JONATHAN BERENT, A.C.S.W.
Author of *Beyond Shyness: How to Conquer Social Anxieties*

"This is a fantastic book. Once you pick it up, it is difficult to put down. Livingstone's major premise here is that you can access your higher self while you are exercising. Getting in touch with your higher self allows the reader to face emotional pain without fear and confusion. This book also teaches the reader how to ask questions about their emotional pain. If you know something has been troubling you for a long time and don't know where to start working through it, this book is for you."

—RICK FRISHMAN

Author of *Guerrilla Publicity Networking Magic Author 101 Series*

"*The Body-Mind-Soul Solution* was a revelation to me. As someone who works in one of the sedentary, unsure and difficult professions of writing, I have long found solace in vigorous physical exercise. The hell with solace, I find salvation. Bob Livingstone's book gave me a depth of inspiration and understanding as to why this connection is critical to all of us. If you're stressful and difficult, read this book and get off your ass and start moving."

—JAMES DALESSANDRO

Author of *1906*

"Livingstone's work is innovative and creative. He combines the well researched benefits of physical exercise with self-reflection. His writing style is highly entertaining. The case examples help the reader gain important insights into their emotional lives. I highly recommend this book."

—LAURA L. SMITH, PH.D.

Author of *Anxiety and Depression Workbook for Dummies, Depression for Dummies,* and *Overcoming Anxiety for Dummies*

"Bob Livingstone addresses both mind and body fitness in this unique and enjoyable book. *The Body-Mind-Soul Solution* is gentle, uncomplicated, and very easy to use. Anyone who exercises can put the time to good use by uncovering and dealing with emotional pain at the same time."

—GLORIA ARENSON, MS, MFT
Author of *Five Simple Steps to Emotional Healing*

"Do you want to deal with overwhelming feelings and memories? Do you want to do it in a way that produces calm control, strength, increased self-confidence, and well-being? Then Bob Livingstone's book is precisely what you need . . . and want. He provides you with simple ways to move through stuck grief, death of a loved one, healing the teenager within, anger that hurts the ones you love, and ancestor (race/ethnic) anguish. Using detailed case studies, he shows how individuals exercised and questioned their way through their pain. The combination of exercise and self-help techniques is brilliant because increasingly the medical establishment is recognizing the benefits of exercise for emotional problems, such as anxiety and depression. Through his program, you can simultaneously make yourself more physically and psychologically fit. If you want to face your emotional pain without fear and confusion and grow personally as well, don't just read this book . . . live it!"

—SIGNE A. DAYHOFF, PH.D.

"Bob Livingstone truly understands the connection between mind and body and has created a breakthrough work in *The Body-Mind-Soul Solution*. This easy to read book creatively combines self-help techniques with physical exercise to promote emotional healing and growth. If you are looking for a means to heal from the death of a loved one, the end of a relationship, or other intense personal loss, this book is for you."

—DR. TIM URSINY

Author of *The Coward's Guide to Conflict, The Coach's Handbook* and *The Confidence Plan: How to Build a Stronger You*

"Bob Livingstone has given us a seriously excellent way of working through trauma with those who find it exceptionally difficult. I have used his ideas very successfully with many clients, especially with those who seem repeatedly to get stuck, those with intimate shame/rage issues stemming from harsh experience, and those who have a history of quietly "winding up" to rages. I have seen clients with brain injury and reduced executive control carry themselves through crisis by facing their pain with the kind of exercise that works best for them. I suspect his observations may work well for most of us, clients and clinicians alike."

—PAT POTTER-EFRON

"This is an important book whose time has come. *The Body-Mind-Soul Solution* reminds us that exercise is important, not just for our physical well-being, but is a crucial component of our emotional and mental well-being. In this book you'll learn to maximize your workout time by uncovering the source of emotional pain and learning to heal and recover from the issues that keep you from true health and peace. Your exercise program will now have a whole new purpose and import in your life. I highly recommend this book for anyone who wants to feel great on every level, body, mind and spirit."

—KATHERINE DREYER

Author of *ChiRunning: A Revolutionary Approach to Effortless and Injury-free Running* and *ChiWalking: Five Mindful Steps to Lifelong Health and Energy*

THE BODY MIND SOUL SOLUTION

Healing Emotional Pain through Exercise

BOB LIVINGSTONE

PEGASUS BOOKS
NEW YORK

The Body-Mind-Soul Solution

Pegasus Books LLC
45 Wall Street, Suite 1021
New York, NY 10005

Library of Congress Cataloging-in-Publication Data is available.

ISBN: 978-1-933648-54-5

10 9 8 7 8 6 5 4 3 2 1

Printed in the United States of America
Distributed by Consortium

Dedicated to the loving memory of my mother
Barbara Livingstone 1921–2006

Table of Contents

Acknowledgements

I would like to give heartfelt thanks to: Claiborne Hancock, Publisher of Pegasus Books, for giving me the opportunity of a lifetime. Editor extraordinaire and mentor Lou Aronica, for his skills, which are nothing less than magical. Peter Skutches for his meticulous line editing; who made a strong book an even bolder one. My family and friends for their love and support: Ruth Samsel, Marion Livingstone, Kevin, Alex, and Rachel Stone, Linda Camarena, Othello and Yolanda Meadows, Sharon and Norman Kman, Wayne Veidt, Kathy Carlson, Moby Coquillard, Toni DeMarco, Karen Lindahl, Al Ferrer, Fred Pecker, Susan Solomon, Akinyele Sadiq, Sue Mailhot, Ken Shure, Liv Rockefeller, David Spero, Aisha Kassahoun, Ron Veronda, Denise Hulett, Rev. Linda Siddall and the staff of Magic Sports/Runner's Feet, Karen Johnson and Marcus Book Store, Rafat Haddad and 3 Bees Coffee, Rene Walker, Derethia Duval, Robert Badame, and Sarah Russell. The case study participants, for sharing their lives with me. Most of all, my wife, Gail Meadows, who has stood by me through thick and thin.

Introduction
How I Discovered This Innovative Program

I was suffering, but I didn't know why. I was fearful I'd return to a constant state of feeling nothing at all. I was afraid I'd slip back into the numbness—a place where sadness and anger are impossible to experience; where pain is neither processed nor acknowledged; where joy is viewed as some cruel, cosmic joke. I feared I was going to free fall into the numbness and never escape. It was like being mired in quicksand. It was getting more and more difficult to breathe.

I had lived much of my life in this awful condition. It began when my father died, when I was fifteen years old, and continued until I was forty. The numbness led me to such self-destructive behavior as drug abuse and terrible feelings of self-loathing. As I entered midlife, however, I began my own psychotherapy treatment and learned how to step out and away from the numbness. I also wrote *Redemption of the Shattered: A Teenager's Healing*

1

Journey through Sandtray Therapy. Finally, after twenty-five years of anguish, I was able to enjoy extended periods of genuine happiness through writing.

But something ominous happened when I turned fifty-one. I began drifting into the numbness again. I recognized its telltale signs—the grip of the insensate despair, the large doses of confusion—and it was wearing me down. My neck hurt and I seemed to have a sinus headache every day, the kind where the throbbing starts just beneath the eye and the pain radiates throughout the brain.

In the moments when I could actually think clearly, I attempted to understand the reasons why I was again being besieged by despair. At this point in my career, I was deeply involved in promoting *Redemption* and frequently stayed up most of the night banging away at the computer. I recognized that I felt overwhelming pressure to succeed as a writer, but I didn't understand why this need for success had become so consuming. At the same time, I was working with a number of teenage clients in my psychotherapy practice, and their angst regularly triggered my own ugly adolescent memories.

Among these memories, two were exceptionally vivid. One was of my fifth-grade teacher telling me that I was the dumbest student she'd had in forty years of teaching. The other was of my ninth-grade guidance counselor telling me in front of my parents that, based on the results of a set of standardized tests, I was not smart enough to go to college and recommending I should enroll in vocational classes. I took college prep courses despite her recommendations and proceeded to fail most of them because deep down inside I believed she was right.

Three decades later, in the midst of my despair, I focused again on these deflating events. Perhaps if I were a successful, best-selling author, my fifth-grade teacher and ninth-grade guidance counselor would apologize to me on national television, maybe on Oprah. Perhaps the world would then view me as a smart person. I could understand why their dismissal of my intelligence and capabilities galled me, but I couldn't understand why I was still so desperate for redemption from their judgments. After all, these people had long been out of my life.

Many of my teenage clients had problems with drug use. At times in my sessions with them memories of my own drug abuse would kick in and I would readily relate to their struggles. Often, though, I'd go beyond empathy; I'd feel as if I myself was still living in a state of teenage angst with these issues left still unresolved for me. It seemed that somehow I could not let go of my own adolescence. On one hand, I wanted to leave it all behind me, but on the other hand, I clung to those memories embedded deep in my heart as if I'd never let them go. Why?

My father died abruptly. I was fifteen. It was the greatest loss of my life. Yet, I had been able, years later, to get in touch with my feelings about his death and grieve his loss. I documented this long journey in my first book. After I finished it, I took time to think about his life in terms of my father himself as opposed to only processing the effects of his death on me. The saddest fact of his life was that he'd never had the opportunity to realize his dream of owning a small business. For some reason the fact of my father's unfulfilled dream continued to be upsetting to me, but I couldn't figure out why.

He died at the age of fifty-six. Actually, I did not know how old he really was until I read the short obituary in the newspaper. I had thought he was in his early forties: My mother and father felt there was a stigma in the 1960's about having a parent that was too old, so my parents fabricated his birth date. They worried that the other kids and perhaps adults in my hometown would look down on me because I had a father who was older than the other dads of kids my age.

When I turned fifty, I began worrying that I would die by the time I was fifty-six. If I experienced some new physical pain, I immediately imagined it might be a disease, despite the fact that I was very athletic and ate a healthy and balanced diet, unlike my father, who died of a stroke. Why was I dwelling on my own mortality so much?

I spent an incredible amount of time reflecting on these plaguing issues. I felt like a dog chasing its tail, however, going around in circles and getting absolutely nowhere. I sensed that something deeper lay underneath these issues, something that I needed to face for my life to become more joyful. But still I remained numb, and every day I'd think about my father, his death, the teenagers in therapy, my own adolescence, my mortality until exhaustion forced me into a fitful, unsatisfying sleep.

Then one day I found a new way to face my emotional pain.

I awoke from one of those truncated sleeps and stumbled across the bedroom to where my running clothes hung. I slowly put them on in the early morning darkness. I was sleep-deprived, my body ached from sleeping at a bad angle, and my head was beating with a sinus flare-up. I really needed to work out.

I put Mary J Blige's *Dance for Me* album on my MP3 player. I really wanted to absorb its energy. As I began my five-mile run, with the music flowing into my ears, I started thinking about everything that was bothering me. I silently asked myself, "What is upsetting me right now?" But I did not press myself for an answer. I simply found my running rhythm and allowed patience to rule the hour.

The answer came suddenly, in the form of a memory.

A recollection of a happier time several years before flashed upon my mind. My wife and I had been taking care of a little girl, Laura, on weekends and on vacations. She had always seemed to be connected to me spiritually, and I recalled the fun we had together laughing and listening to music. I enjoyed reading to her at night and teaching her how to read, cook, play sports and behave in good restaurants. At that moment of recollection I realized how much I really loved that little girl. We'd been helping her aunt raise her, but one day her aunt had a falling-out with us over a disagreement on her child-rearing methods and we were never allowed to take care of her again. The door was shut in our face and there was nothing we could do about it. The pain of this remembered loss took away my breath as I continued running. The tears that streamed down my face mixed with the sweat that flowed from my pores.

Once the run was over, I was pleased that I was able to connect with my feelings surrounding the loss of Laura. I was also surprised that this loss still affected me so deeply, for I thought I had worked through this problem. I had no idea it still troubled me. Then I wondered if possibly, the combination of exercise and self-examination over what was troubling me had allowed the blocked feelings to surface.

After the workout was over, I dried off without taking a shower because I wanted to I write down my thoughts and feelings immediately. I want to be sure not to forget anything. I continued to make journal entries after each of my runs but I found it impossible to remember every thought and feeling that I experienced while I was working out. So I purchased a small digital voice recorder that I could utilize as I ran. What a vision from technological hell I'd become: running while talking into a recorder while listening to an MP3 player.

During the early stages of this process, as I continued to grieve the loss of Laura, I found myself getting in touch with unresolved issues from my adolescence, and I connected to my feelings about father's abruptly shortened life in a new way. On reviewing my initial series of journal entries, I realized that I had indeed discovered a new mode of self-help therapy based on merging the main principle of psychotherapy—asking questions about what is troubling you—with the mental health benefits of physical exercise. My journal entries revealed a step-by-step process by which to face and deal with emotional pain. Bolstered by my discovery, I became confident that any person might grapple successfully with emotional pain this same way. Once the pain is faced, it can then possibly be resolved.

There is no quick fix to resolving emotional pain. However, this program can teach you how to deal with your emotional pain in a calm, thoughtful, nonthreatening manner that enables you first to face it, then to chip away at its frightening elements, and finally begin to look at ways to resolve it. You are likely, nonetheless, to experience surprising revelations during your very first exercise session.

The Body-Mind-Soul Solution will teach you how to connect with your higher self. Some call this higher self the soul, the residence of wisdom or a place of spirituality. Others find in the higher self their connection with God. Exercise in itself elevates you to a calm reflective state. Exercise combined with self questioning as regards emotional pain can bond to the healing power of the higher self. The wedding of the mind and body to the higher place will provide reassuring answers to these painful questions. You will discover, too, that you can retain and enjoy this connection to your higher self for a longer period of time while you are exercising than when you're at rest. The changes in brain chemistry that occur while exercising can explain scientifically why this state of reflective and receptive calmness is induced. But there is also the magic of the experience that transpires when you combine exercise and self-questioning. You may have been emotionally "stuck" for many years, and suddenly, in a revelatory flash, you feel hopeful that your life can change. As you begin to understand why you have been stuck, you will develop ways to move on. You will be renewed. There is something like magic in that, too.

My discovery of the Body-Mind-Soul Solution was either a happy accident or the fulfillment of my personal destiny. I believe it will be of tremendous benefit to you and it will help you discover a serenity you've never before known.

Chapter One
Emotional Pain

Emotional pain is the hurt that's caused by a distressing event or events in your life. You may be unaware of this pain, or you may be conscious of it, but have no idea which events or memories triggered it. You may sense that something is wrong but not know what the something is, or you may have a clear understanding of what's causing the hurt inside yourself but are fearful of addressing it. You may experience emotional pain as a physical ailment such as a digestive problem, tightness in the neck or shoulder muscles, a skin problem, or chronic tiredness. The pain also prompts unpleasant memories that cause you to feel afraid, sad, angry, unresolved, or stuck.

In the Body-Mind-Soul Solution, you focus upon a specific kind of emotional pain and ask questions about its source and ramifications while you are exercising. In order to face your anguish, you need to be able to first define the kind of emotional pain you are experiencing. In my almost twenty years of clinical work, I have identified five major types of emotional pain. Each is described below.

STUCK GRIEF

If you have experienced the death of a loved one a year or more ago and feel that the loss happened yesterday, you may be a victim of stuck grief. If your boyfriend broke up with you six months ago and you still think about him all the time, you may be experiencing stuck grief. If you are a young or middle-aged person and find that you spend much more time dwelling on past memories than focusing on the present, you may be suffering from stuck grief.

People who suffer the effects of stuck grief experience an absence of emotion. They have difficulty accessing anger, sadness, passion or join in anything. They are so emotionally limited that they are unaware of being stuck let alone being clear as to why.

I led a bereavement-recovery group through a hospice organization for nine years. The group met once a week for an hour and a half. It was open to anyone who had recently lost a loved one through death. Some of the group members attended only a few sessions, while others showed up every week for a year or more. Many of them were able to move through the five different stages of grief, which, according to Elisabeth Kübler-Ross, are denial, depression, anger, bargaining, and acceptance. Some were not: They were stuck. They resisted moving on with their lives because they were afraid of what might happen if they let go of their deceased loved one. They feared starting new relationships, finding other support systems, and developing new interests.

Mired in the past, members of the group viewed the future as dismal. Their goal was to simply get through each day with as little upheaval as possible. They firmly believed that regaining any sort of happiness not only was impossible but also wrong because to feel happy was to be disloyal to their dear departed loved ones. Daily cemetery visits, filling "shrines" with their loved ones' pictures, and extended discussions about the past were both rituals that epitomized their stuck grief and activities that imprisoned them in its misery. Behavior of this sort is neither unusual nor harmful shortly after the death of someone close to you. If it continues for an extended period, however, serious psychological problems arise.

I have worked with several clients who have had similar experiences when dealing with the end of a romantic relationship. Although their former partners have made it abundantly clear the relationship is over, the clients refuse to believe it has ended. Instead of acknowledging fact, they ask me for tips on how to win the other person back. This willful inability to let go of a relationship can continue for months or longer. Meanwhile, their lives remain on hold.

People who experience stuck grief are in denial and do not realize it. Convinced that the time spent with their lost or departed loved ones comprised the very best part of their lives, they can conceive of nothing that could even begin to duplicate that rich sense of fulfillment. The future thus becomes not worth living.

The first step in dealing with stuck grief is to acknowledge that you are in denial. The next step is to grieve the loss by

experiencing the anger, sadness, and sense of abandonment attached to it. If you can break through denial and face the pain, you
will be able to begin to let go of the past and begin to move on.

THE DEATH OF A LOVED ONE

All of us will experience the death of someone close to us, and it
is normal to grieve this loss. This form of emotional pain differs
from stuck grief. Those experiencing stuck grief tend to not feel
or express their deep feelings about the loss while others begin
grieving immediately.

Still, it is never easy to deal with such grief, and unresolved
issues can complicate it. You may feel that you did not have the
opportunity to say good-bye or did not say to your loved one
all that you wanted before she or he died. At first, you may be
in shock and feel numb. Later, sadness may overwhelm you. You
may cry out deep guttural sounds and touch on a deep, sad place
inside you that you didn't know existed.

I have worked extensively with clients who experience this
form of emotional pain. I know that nothing I say can take their
pain away and the most healing aid I can offer is to listen. For by
talking, they will begin to deal with the pain.

THE TEENAGER WITHIN

We all have within us a teenager who has lived through identity
confusion, mood swings, passionate opinions and relationship

angst. I have worked with adult clients who have not successfully mastered social skills they should have mastered during adolescence. They have difficulty maintaining relationships, which are characterized by continuous arguing, intermittent breakups, tearful reunions, and dramatic flare-ups. People trapped in such relationships will often involve their family members and friends in the most intimate details of their private lives in an effort to line up support for their "side." Impulsive behavior—such as calling your girlfriend every hour on the hour beginning at two in the morning—is common.

The erratic behavior of such people commonly extends to their performance at the workplace. They often move from one job to another in an endless search for an undefined sense of fulfillment. They frequently have issues with bosses and other authority figures, and when they are reprimanded for being disrespectful, they fail to learn from their mistakes.

While this kind of behavior is typical of teenage angst, it becomes troublesome in an adult. In all likelihood, an adult who demonstrates behavior more typical of an adolescent has important issues that were not resolved during his or her younger years: parental physical abuse or neglect, clashes with authority figures, lack of guidance from parents on how to deal with intense emotions, ostracism by peers and feelings of inadequacy, of never measuring up to expectations. Facing the emotional pain surrounding behavior that originates in these issues is the first step toward resolution.

THE ANGER THAT HURTS
THOSE WE LOVE

If you make hurtful comments to those close to you and have a temper that is right below the surface of your civility and that can be triggered at any moment, you may suffer from misplaced and misdirected anger that causes both you and your loved one emotional distress. This is especially true if you continue to feel remorseful after each new hurtful episode, but have failed to make any progress in improving your behavior.

Healing the anger that hurts those you love requires that you take responsibility for your words and not blame others for your behavior. A couple of years ago, I co-led a group for men who physically and/or verbally battered their partners. The group, participants court-mandated, met over a fifty-two-week period. During discussions of their issues, it was very common for one of the members to say, "If she didn't fill-in-the-blank, I never would have hit her. She needs to control her actions so I won't beat her again."

I ask my clients with anger management issues to pay attention to what their body is feeling. I ask them where they carry stress in their bodies. I ask them to check in with their brains and pay close attention to what they are thinking. Being tuned in to what is going on inside the mind and the body can help reduce this type of emotional pain considerably.

ANCESTORS' ANGUISH

Many of us have ancestors who were victims of genocide, torture, and slavery and some people feel this ancestral pain on a deeply personal level. For example, if you are Jewish and worry constantly that you might be taken away in the middle of the night, you are probably identifying with ancestors murdered in the Holocaust. If you are African-American and fear you'll be forced to work for no pay, or be physically beaten and raped, you may be closely connected to ancestors who were slaves.

The healing goal here is to not to undo history, but to understand how our ancestors' anguish affects us today and how we can channel our bitterness, rage, and fear into some positive force—to find ways to heal ourselves, our families, our towns, our countries, and our world.

I have worked with a number of clients who were victims of racial discrimination. Some of the emotional effects of the racism they suffered are distrust of others, low self-esteem, hyper-vigilance, depression, anxiety, and overwhelming fear. My first goal as a therapist is to recognize racism itself as a mental disorder and honor those victims of it who come into my office. It has been my experience that when clients begin to process how this hatred affects them, they get in touch with the cruelties and suffering their ancestors endured. In this awareness they find solace and strength.

These five types of emotional pain can be debilitating. They can all, however, be faced through the Body-Mind-Soul Solution. The benefits of doing so are considerable, as the next chapter will show . . .

Chapter Two
The Eight Benefits of
Facing Your Emotional Pain

The Body-Mind Soul Solution helps you to face your emotional pain. Doing so is extremely liberating, for it allows you to move on with your life. Over the course of my clinical work, I have identified the following eight primary benefits in facing your emotional pain.

UNDERSTANDING THE CAUSE OF YOUR PAIN

If you can understand what is causing your pain, you have a much better chance of some day letting it go. You may discover, too, that the source of the distress was creating other problems in your life, which will also diminish as a result.

Ralph G. is fifty, married with three children, and is a successful businessman living in a wealthy suburb. When he walked into my office several years ago, he was clearly troubled. He was unsure if his father, who had died four years earlier after a long bout with cancer, actually loved him. An alcoholic, his father had never shared with him any feelings of joy, sadness, or inadequacy.

Ralph was suffering from insomnia, was anxiety-ridden, and was uncertain about the direction he wanted to take at this point in his life. He anxiously shared with me the most important story of his childhood. His father had worked hard all his life to achieve financial security. A banker, he had in time accumulated enough money to afford his family a sizeable house in a prestigious neighborhood. Then one day his father made a financial decision that ended up nearly bankrupting the family. When Ralph was ten years old, they moved from their mansion to a tract house, where they survived on food stamps.

Ralph's father never recovered from this economic slide into lower-class living. Denied access to all facets of his former life, he essentially withdrew from reality. He anesthetized his pain with alcohol. He never admitted that he had made a terrible mistake, and by unwritten rule this defining catastrophic event was never to be discussed. Ralph's mother supported her husband in this abject denial.

Ralph learned in therapy that this denial had from the outset caused him deep emotional angst. He was the only member of the family ever to express worry or concern that things were going badly.

Whenever he did, though, the rest of his household either ignored him or sneered at him. Rebuffed, Ralph in his teens cut himself off from his family and strove to become self-sufficient; as a result, he learned not to trust adults or anyone else. He believed that he could rely only on himself. As an adult, Ralph spent much of his time looking into the future and worrying that he was not meeting his goals. If a business plan went awry, he either panicked or became enraged.

At first, Ralph was resistant to confronting the source of his emotional pain. After several sessions, though, he had an epiphany. He came to understand that each time he encountered a problem, he became fearful that he was going to fail the way his father had done. In the midst of this panic, he would imagine losing all he had gained: his material goods as well as his wife and children. In time, Ralph accepted that it was impossible for all plans to play out exactly as you visualize them. He also came to accept that he was not perfect and that he did not have to be infallible.

He then began to focus on his feelings toward his father and his father's connection to him. Ralph's father never praised his son's accomplishments or offered him any suggestions for self-improvement in school. Ralph was a good athlete, but his father never attended any of his sporting events. Nor could Ralph remember that his dad had ever demonstrated any affection toward him, or engaged in any sports or board games with him. Ralph recalled that he had taken an interest in science only because he felt that through it he might be able to connect with his father. As it turned out, science was the only interest they in any way shared.

Throughout his therapy Ralph strove to find the truth about what lay in his father's heart, in an attempt to establish an emotional and spiritual connection with him. Focusing on childhood memories, Ralph searched his mind, heart, and soul in the hope of discovering some glimpse of tenderness he'd received from his dad. Sadly, he never succeeded. Ralph came to understand that his father's parents were themselves cold people who had never shown their son how to care for others.

Gradually Ralph became less preoccupied with his quest. He realized that the love he was desperately searching for would never come, and so he chose to find that love somewhere else. He stopped looking outside of himself for affirmation and began to look for strength within. He found it, too. He discovered that he could calm himself when he panicked and turn despair into hope. He learned to live in the moment with his wife and children, and he was able to say good-bye to his dad.

By understanding what caused his emotional pain, he was able to leave it behind.

EXPERIENCING PERSONAL GROWTH

An experience as dramatic as facing your emotional pain can create significant personal growth by increasing self-knowledge and insight. With this growth might come an increased sense of spirituality, a belief in your capacity to change dramatically, and a continually evolving compassion for others.

Jane M. is twenty-eight-year-old woman who was referred to me because she was being physically and verbally abused by her husband. My initial impression was that she was quite nervous and had difficulty organizing her thoughts. However, once she became comfortable being with me, she had a harrowing story to tell.

She had been married for four months when her husband, previously a kind and considerate man, began hitting her. He would yell at her too and at her four-year-old daughter from a previous marriage, a child he allowed his friends to physically and verbally abuse. One night he accused Jane of cheating on him, and when she denied it, he started slapping her in the face and then began punching her. He knocked out one of her teeth. She called the police, who responded by taking her husband to jail.

That night she packed her clothes and gathered up her daughter. They moved to her aunt's house in another town: a temporary arrangement until she was able to find her own housing. However, her aunt was a methamphetamine addict who experienced frequent mood swings, and soon Jane and her daughter found themselves on the street again. A series of contacts had eventually led her to the local battered women's shelter where Jane and her daughter were residing when she found her way to my office.

For the first time in ages, Jane could let down her guard a little bit. She started therapy and began to experience personal growth. Revealing that this was not the first abusive relationship she had been in, she expressed her need to understand why she was attracted to violent men. She read articles about domestic violence and realized that she was suffering from Battered Women's Syndrome. She realized, too, the fallacy of blaming herself for the beatings; she learned to put the responsibility on the men who beat her.

Jane continued to grow as she plumbed her family's considerable history of violence. She had witnessed her father beating her mother and she learned that it is common for women to be attracted to men like their fathers, even if they find physical abuse totally abhorrent. Now Jane knows that she was attracted to her husband because his behavior, belief system, and mannerisms echoed her father's. She has learned to recognize the "red flags" of potentially dangerous partners; she has made a commitment to live a nonviolent life.

She has truly grown into a more fulfilling life.

REDUCING THE INFLUENCE THAT EMOTIONAL PAIN HAS ON YOUR LIFE

Denying emotional pain can be hazardous to your mental and physical health. Freeing yourself from the chains of a chronic internal ache can be liberating. The energy previously spent focusing on obstructive hurt can now be utilized for increased creative and financial productivity.

Elaine G. was overwhelmed with emotional pain when she entered my office for the first time. In the midst of a nerve-racking divorce, she was worried about how her three children were dealing with its fallout. She herself was experiencing panic attacks. She'd become increasingly fearful of traveling anywhere on her own.

Elaine, born in Louisiana, was one of four siblings. Because her quite wealthy parents were away from home much of the time while she was growing up, her primary caretakers were nannies who made sure that all her basic needs were met.

It seemed that Elaine's parents did not know how to interact with her. They encouraged achievement and material success, but they did not teach their daughter how to deal with fear, loneliness, and isolation. It was up to the hired help to soothe her when she became upset. Aware that Elaine became panicky when she was left alone, they made sure that she never was. This panic and rescuing pattern began as soon as she was born and continued until her favorite nanny died when Elaine was seventeen. It proved to be psychologically paralyzing for Elaine, for she never learned how to utilize her own internal resources in order to face emotional pain.

Now, at age thirty-eight, she was afraid to go anywhere alone and more convinced than concerned that she could not take care of herself. She would go into full panic mode when she was driving in desolate, rural areas. At the peak of this alarming phase, she felt that everyone on earth had abandoned her and that she was destined to live entirely by herself for all time.

Working with me, Elaine began to accept that her parents' neglect had really harmed her, and this admission helped her to stop blaming herself for her difficulties. She realized that her parents had never seen her as a little girl, teenager, or young woman, but rather as an entity who was a good student, a strong athlete, an attractive fashion model—attributes she had developed in order to obtain her parents' approval. She felt that her mother in particular viewed these achievements as a means to increase her status among New Orleans upper-class society.

In therapy, Elaine examined the reasons for her panic and worked diligently to overcome them. She came to understand that she had not experienced the developmental stage in which a child masters self-soothing and learns to deal with fear when it strikes. She now was discovering what she had missed and relished this new knowledge. She also was able to break her family's cycle of parental neglect by bonding with her children in a healthy way and seeing them as not as objects to admire but human beings to love.

By reducing the influence her emotional pain had placed on her soul, she has given herself a new life.

DECREASING STRESS AND INCREASING SELF-ESTEEM

If you are denying emotional anguish, day-to-day life is filled with pressure. When stress becomes a constant, restlessness and sleep problems occur; you become jumpy and maybe alterably overly aggressive or extremely passive. Everything becomes a series of crises, and your movement from one crisis to the next defines your lifestyle.

When Frank M, a fifty-five-year-old man, first consulted me, he said that he suffered from low self-esteem and that at times the stress he felt would cause him to either erupt in rage or withdraw from everyone close to him. Because he was living alone, he also often experienced feelings of isolation and intense loneliness. Frank described his father, an alcoholic who had recently became clean and sober without the support of AA or any other program, as a rigid man who was always extremely demanding of his son though Frank was never sure exactly what his father wanted from him. When he drank, his dad became verbally abusive and he would berate Frank's mother and his two older brothers. Frank has no memories of his father praising or encouraging him. If Frank was too tired or ill to give his all to an effort, his father would tell him to "suck it up" and move on.

Frank had risen to upper management in the airline industry, and, while he felt that he was good at his job, he heard a constantly punitive voice inside him telling him that he would never measure up, no matter what he did. His intimate relationships, too, were fraught with problems. Potential partners accused him of being emotionally distant because he did not share personal feelings. Feeling that he was totally responsible for his partner's happiness and fearing that he would fail, he walled up his emotions. He also believed, not surprisingly, that anything that went wrong in his relationships had to be his fault. Frank lived in the land of self-loathing and endless stress. He was plagued by apathy. Once athletic, he now engaged in virtually no physical activity.

Over time, Frank realized that the negative, punishing voice he kept hearing was not his own; it was his father's. Indeed, the major lesson he obtained from his dad was how to be harsh on himself and others. Frank realized, too, that he could not only change his negative thinking process, he could also change the way he felt about himself. He learned to let his father's "voice" go, and whenever a crisis at work came up, instead of blaming himself for the predicament, he would methodically problem-solve. He learned to treat himself better, and he began exercising.

He is currently involved in a positive relationship with a woman. He now feels free to share his feelings of joy and disappointment with the relationship.

The energy once devoted to the stress of emotional pain, he can now apply to much more productive pursuits.

IMPROVING YOUR RELATIONSHIPS WITH OTHERS

If you deny emotional pain, your relationships with others can range from the indifferent to the superficial to the antagonistic. It is impossible to have a relationship based on mutuality, respect, love, or genuineness, if you aren't able to face what is troubling you.

James K. was in his late thirties when he reached a pivotal point in his life. He had been married ten years and had two young children, but the family was not functioning well. One day his wife gave him an ultimatum: "Stop being verbally abusive toward me and the children or I will file for divorce." James took his wife's directive seriously and embarked on a difficult journey.

James has a high-pressure sales and management position requiring him to work as many as eighty hours a week: A heavy workload that makes it very difficult for him to spend quality time with his family. I sensed that, while James was highly driven and knew how to succeed in the corporate world, he had next to no knowledge about how to interact constructively with his family. He tended to view the world from an intellectual perspective. For example, if he played soccer with his five-year-old son for a half hour, the two of them simply kicking the ball back and forth, the fact that the play seemed to have no purpose, no soccer drills, no preparation for games, bothered James. He had a hard time just being with his son and enjoying the moment.

His demanding work responsibilities led to daily stress that started from the moment James awoke. If his wife was too slow in preparing breakfast or if his two-year-old daughter took too long to dress in the morning, James would lose all patience and unleash a loud emotional outburst. His face would turn beet red and he yelled at his family, and often some of the words he chose proved to be extremely hurtful. The effects of these outbursts on the family required a significant healing period.

Usually when one spouse forces another into therapy, the partner that attends the sessions does not take it seriously, because he does not really believe he has a problem. This was not the case with James, however. He attended therapy on a regular basis despite his heavy work schedule. It was my impression that he did so out of remorse: He felt tremendously guilty after his verbal outbursts and he truly did not want to lose his family. Wondering why he lashed out so angrily with his family when he was stressed, James began to uncover the source of his fury early on in his therapy.

It turned out that his father had left his mother when he was five years old. He'd moved a couple of hundred miles away and never thereafter bothered to get in touch with his son. James never understood why he was abandoned and developed a strategy to deal with the fact of it. He'd simply dismiss it by saying to himself, "That's just the way it was and I have to go on living my life." Pushing down the emotional pain, though, caused James to direct his anger at the wrong people.

Working with me, he began journaling and purposely watching movies that triggered an emotional response. As he began to plumb the depths of his loss, he was, to his relief, able to attach his anger to actual memories—that of his father deserting him, his older brother, and that of his mother and of his mother passing out from the exhaustion of working two jobs in order to make ends meet because his father never paid child support.

James decided to contact his father with the purpose of meeting with him. James wanted to confront him about his desertion, and he wrote down what he wanted to say. He called up additional memories of not having a father's guidance, support, or presence; feeling discarded; and in doing so, James realized that he wanted to be the antithesis of his biological father. He really wanted to have a close relationship with his children, and whereas he had once dreaded contact with them, he now looked forward to spending time with them, having fun, and watching them grow.

James's relationship with his wife also improved as he became more empathetic toward her and more fully aware of how much he really loved her.

Once James faced his emotional pain, the most important relationships in his life improved dramatically.

TRANSFORMING UNHAPPINESS TO JOY

When you deny emotional pain, you spend a lot of time feeling unhappy. If you confront your anguish, you will be able to experience a level of joy, happiness, and excitement that has been missing from your life.

Doug M., an active participant in Alcoholics Anonymous, had been clean and sober for more than fifteen years. A tri-athlete who performed well in his age division, he strived to exercise regularly. When I met him, he was a single forty-one-year-old man who owned a roofing company. During our first session, Doug complained of being generally dissatisfied and bored with life. At times he felt that he was merely going through the motions.

The main source of Doug's discontentment was his relationship with his live-in partner, Julie. They had been living together for about five years when he began an affair with another woman. Doug was not clear how he felt about either woman, but he was certain that his involvement in a second relationship was not solving his problems. Rather, it was compounding the confusion.

Doug's parents had never discussed how they worked their way through conflicts, and therefore Doug never learned to discuss his feelings. He realized that not facing his problems, as he was now doing, was a primary reason for his alcoholism, although he did not think he was in danger of returning to drinking. He realized, too, that he did not talk about much of anything that truly mattered with Julie. Doug recognized his pattern: He got involved with women who admired him and he did not question his feelings for them as long as he was attracted to them physically. He began to see that his intimate relationships were not really intimate at all. They were in fact the symptoms of another addiction, his need to be admired and placed on a pedestal.

Although Doug did not uncover the reason for his pain in our sessions together, he accepted that he had established this particular pattern, and he was determined to break it. He broke up with the woman with whom he was having the affair by being honest. He told her the affair was not in his best interests and that he needed to work on his relationship with Julie. Feeling quite relieved and empowered after the breakup, he decided to risk sharing his true feelings with Julie. He let her know that he was unhappy with their relationship, that he felt they did not seem to have much in common, that he had grown distant from her. A few weeks later they agreed to break up, and Julie moved out.

Doug began to live alone for really the first time in his life. He paid attention to the ups and downs life offered in a way he never had before. He experienced fulfillment from his job and his sport. Instead of pushing his emotions away, he permitted his feelings to run free. When he ended therapy, he was enjoying life and looking forward to the day when he could find a true soul mate.

By facing his emotional pain, even though he had not uncovered its source, he had allowed himself to be happy.

DEVELOPING NEW COPING SKILLS TO IMPROVE YOUR QUALITY OF LIFE

Once you face your emotional pain, you can learn to cope with life in new ways. Developing new coping skills requires time and practice. Such skills do not come naturally at first, but eventually they become integrated into your daily routine. The new coping skill you first need to develop is to notice the signals that you are about to become depressed, anxious, angry, or other wise unsettled in a way that will have a negative impact on your ability to lead a contented life.

James's life floundered in turmoil when he became verbally abusive to his wife and kids. Not until he was in therapy was he aware of what actually was happening to him before, during, and after one of these blow-ups. Eventually he learned that his anger was brewing long before he began yelling out, that actually he'd become agitated as soon as he woke up in the morning because he was overwhelmed with the work he had to complete by nightfall. If any of his family members interfered with the process of his agenda, he would start shouting. He learned to tell himself that his family was not going to perform perfectly and complete all their morning tasks in a timely fashion. If he was late getting to his morning meeting, then he was late; no big deal. He also became aware that another emotion came into play before he felt rage. When his children or wife fell behind schedule, he felt hurt. He felt unloved by them because they were not cooperating. He would say to himself, "Don't they understand that I am working so hard to provide a great life for them? Can't they show their appreciation by getting ready on time?"

James discovered that his expectations were unrealistic. He also learned that just because his family was not prompt did not mean they didn't love him. He learned to be more patient over time by paying attention to his internal signals.

The next coping skill to learn is to distance yourself from the pain. This is different from unhealthy denial of the pain altogether. Rather, it is a coping skill that enables you to deal with the pain when it becomes too much to bear.

Elaine suffered from panic attacks and at times would feel flooded by emotion while experiencing its pain. In such circumstances it was preferable to distance herself from the anguish in order to regroup. For instance, she would engage in a relaxing activity, like taking a warm bath. If she was with friends, she would concentrate on the words the other persons were saying in order to stay connected to the conversation. If she went for a walk, she would focus on the beauty of the sunset or the salty smell of the ocean. With such diversions she was able to let go of the pain temporarily in a healthy manner. She was also able to live more readily in the present, which is a major goal in therapy.

Another essential coping skill is to realize that you have a choice whether to face your emotional pain or not. In fact, when you reach the point where you have the freedom to think about anything you want, you will understand that you have more control over your thinking process than you previously believed was possible.

Ralph suffered from insomnia for years because he would lie awake at night immersed in fear. He was mostly worried about his future, and his anxiety was debilitating at times. Ralph did not feel that he had any choice but to focus on his worries; he firmly believed that worry was his destiny and the only way to deal with his pain. He realized in therapy that in worrying, he was not really facing his emotional pain; he was merely worrying. He learned that he could choose not to worry, that he could let it go and he himself could determine the time to work on his emotional pain.

A final coping skill is to get in touch with and gain access to the higher self: that place inside you that holds the truths about your life: a place where you can find solitude, redemption, and knowledge.

Frank, like many others, was not aware of his higher self when he started therapy. He spent many of his waking hours beating up on himself for what he considered unforgivable mistakes. He eventually discovered his higher self by peeling away layer after layer of bad memories and examining the causes and effects of his emotional pain. He learned that he was actually a good person, not a failure or a demon. He also learned he could find answers to his dilemmas inside himself. Indeed, his higher self served Frank as the kind, understanding father that he'd never had.

RESOLVING EMOTIONAL PAIN

The confrontation of distressing memories and feelings is a journey filled with upheaval, confusion, brazen insight, intense sadness, bold anger, and unbridled joy. Perhaps the greatest discovery during this ordeal is the energy called love, and you can find it anywhere.

Resolving emotional pain is the final aspect of facing emotional pain. Resolving does not mean forgetting about those that have abused, abandoned, or hurt us. To resolve pain, we need to keep a place in our hearts for the people who have hurt us.

For years after my father died, I felt that he was constantly hovering over me like a dark cloud that was eventually going to turn into a destructive tornado. By working on my emotional pain, I found a way to let go of my father and release him into the sky and heavens above. The dark cloud that had lived with me for twenty-five years dissipated.

Resolving emotional pain usually involves forgiveness. This very personal process ultimately leads to forgiving not just the person perceived as the source of your hurt, but forgiving yourself. I finally forgave myself for being in pain for so long without the means to face it. I forgave myself for beating up on my child and teenager within because I didn't know any better. The loss of my father greatly influenced me in becoming a psychotherapist who deals with loss. His death and life have been the main inspiration for the books I have written.

I was in touch with his spirit when I discovered the Body-Mind-Soul Solution.

Chapter Three

Discovering the Source of Your Emotional Pain

P lease complete the Emotional Pain Questionnaire in order to pinpoint the reasons you feel unfulfilled, unhappy, distressed, or confused. Once you have pinpointed the source of your emotional pain, you will know what questions to ask while exercising.

Emotional Pain Questionnaire

1. Symptoms You Are Currently Experiencing that have been ruled out as physical problems by your physician

Do you get headaches? How often? When do you have them?

Do you have muscle pain? In what part of your body? What does it feel like? Is it chronic?

Do you experience rapid heartbeat? When does this happen and how often?

Do you get stomach aches? When does this happen and how often?

Do you grind your teeth at night? Do you have a sore jaw or headaches as a result of this?

Do you have problems falling asleep or staying asleep? Do you wake up in the middle of the night for a prolonged period? How often does this occur?

Do you lack energy or motivation? How long have you experienced being in this state?

Do you have any other physical symptoms that your doctor has ruled out as being physically based?

2. Present Emotional State

Have you been experiencing suicidal thoughts or feelings? IF SO, YOU SHOULD CONTACT A MENTAL HEALTH PROFESSIONAL IMMEDIATELY.

Are you easily agitated? How long have you experienced being in this state? When does this occur?

Do you have difficulty finding enjoyment in activities that once were pleasurable? How long has this been going on? What are those activities?

Do you have difficulty getting along with others? How long has this been going on?

Do you find yourself crying more often lately? When does this occur?

Do you find yourself having no discernible emotional feelings (numbness)? When does this happen?

Do you find yourself feeling disconnected from others? In what kinds of situations does this occur?

Do you have difficulty thinking clearly? When does this take place?

Do you have difficulty concentrating? When does this happen?

Are you worried much of the time? What do you find yourself worrying about?

Are you currently or have you ever taken prescription medication for depression, anxiety, or any other emotional problem? How does it affect you?

Are you afraid to stand up for yourself? In what kinds of situations does this happen? How does this affect you?

Do you have difficulty giving yourself credit when you have done something well? How does this affect you? When did this most recently occur?

Do you find that your feelings are hurt often and that you do not have the ability to soothe yourself? How does this affect you? When was the last time this happened?

Do you have difficulty trusting others? How does it affect you? When was the last time this occurred?

Do you have problems forgiving others? How does it affect you? When was the last time this occurred?

Do you have problems forgiving yourself? How does it affect you? When was the last time this occurred?

Do you have low self-esteem? How long have you experienced this?

Do you have difficulty making and keeping friendships? How does this affect you?

Do you have difficulty making and keeping intimate relationships? How does this affect you?

Do you sense that something is wrong but have difficulty identifying the problem? Please describe what emotions, memories, and physical symptoms you experience in such a situation.

3. Childhood History

Were you physically abused by your parents or others? Describe what happened.

How did this affect you as a child?

Were you neglected by your parents or others close to you? Describe what happened.

How did this affect you as a child?

Were you emotionally abused by your parents or others? Describe what happened.

How did this affect you as a child?

Were you sexually abused as a child? Describe what happened.

How did this affect you as a child?

Did your parents play with you when you were a child? What activities did you do together? How did this affect you?

What were your parents' expectations of you as a child and as a teenager? How did this affect you?

What were your grades like in school? How did you feel about school?

How did your parents discipline you? How did this affect you?

How did your parents deal with their failures? How did this affect you?

Did your parents praise you for doing well? How did this affect you?

What was the most positive event of your childhood? How did this affect you?

What was the most upsetting/traumatic event of your childhood? How did this affect you?

4. Different Kinds of Emotional Pain

STUCK GRIEF

Have you suffered a loss more than a year ago that you are having difficulty getting through? What thoughts and feelings do you have about this?

Did someone close to you die more than a year ago? Do you find yourself thinking about him or her continually?

Did your primary relationship end more than a year ago? Do you find yourself thinking about him or her continually? Are you having a difficult time accepting that the relationship is over?

Do you believe that you will never recover from your loss? How do you visualize your life in the future?

THE LOSS OF A LOVED ONE

Has someone close to you died recently? Who died and what was it like for you?

Do you feel "raw" inside? Why do you feel that you are in so much pain? What was your relationship like with your loved one?

Are you finding it difficult to work or go to school? How are you dealing with this?

Do you worry that you will never get over this overwhelming sense of grief? What does this feel like?

Are you angry that life seems to go on for others while your loved one is now deceased? How do you deal with this?

THE TEENAGER WITHIN

Is there a great deal of drama in your life? When does this happen?

Do you feel restless much of the time? When does this happen?

Do you find it difficult to be satisfied? When does this happen?

Do you often get into confrontations? When does this happen?

Are you confused much of the time? When does this happen?

THE ANGER THAT HURTS THOSE YOU LOVE

Have you hurt someone so deeply that this person is reluctant to forgive you? What happened?

Do you feel guilt and shame for causing your loved one pain? Why do you feel this way?

Do you feel that you are entitled to verbally hurt a loved one? Why do you feel entitled?

Do you feel that you have little to no control over your actions? Why do you feel this way? What have been the consequences of your actions?

Have you ever physically battered a loved one? When did this happen? How do you feel about your actions? What have you done to change your behavior?

THE ANCESTORS ANGUISH

Have your ancestors been victims of genocide? How do they affect you?

Have your ancestors shared stories of loss? How does this affect you?

Do you feel connected to your ancestors' pain? How does this affect you?

Do you find yourself focusing on a specific period of your ancestors' history? How do you benefit from this?

Do you feel that you have any behaviors or feelings that stem from your ancestors' plight? How do they affect you?

The completion of this questionnaire is an essential component of the Body-Mind-Soul Solution. Your diligent effort in this process illuminates fully the hardships you have faced. After reviewing this survey, you should have a clear understanding of the source of your emotional pain.

You can delve further into the profile of emotional pain that you derive from this survey while reading chapter 4, Investigating Emotional Pain. There you will find insights discovered by the case study participants that will help give you a clearer picture of your emotional pain.

Being totally familiar with the results of your emotional pain questionnaire will enable you to plug readily into the possible questions to ask yourself while exercising as per chapter six, The Body-Mind-Soul Solution.

Finally, the responses to this survey will prepare you for Discoveries, chapter 7. Your comprehension of the origins of your emotional pain is a major steppingstone toward discovering new insights, by learning how to face emotional pain without distraction, how to confront anger and sadness fully, how to find your wisdom, and how to use the power of your imagination.

Chapter Four

Investigating Your Emotional Pain

You have now identified the source of your emotional pain. This chapter offers case studies that show how others have discovered the origins of their pain and how their insights affected their day-to-day lives. (All names and identifying information of the case study participants have been changed to protect their confidentiality.) From them, you will see that insights gained from this process prompt me to asking further pertinent questions while exercising and thereby begin the process of emotional healing.

This chapter will address parental abuse and neglect traumas that have been related to me by clients during the past nineteen years. Left untreated, this type of childhood trauma can adversely affect psychological development, physical well-being, mood, the ability to form friendships and intimate relationships, and the ability to trust others.

Ralph G., the fifty-year-old man we met in chapter 2, was anxious, depressed, and very confused for most of his five decades. At different points in his life, he became so withdrawn from everyday reality that he stayed in bed for days at a time. He thought it was possible that a physical problem was causing his inability to function. However, various physicians found nothing physically wrong with him.

Ralph had difficulty developing friendships. He trusted no one. He was thus very demanding of his wife and children, as he expected them to fill the emptiness he felt within himself. He did not like to be alone, and he was frightened of the unknown. Imposing order over his existence, he exhibited obsessive-compulsive tendencies, such as brushing his teeth the same way each day and arranging his desk so that all his pens, pencils, and other stationery items were perfectly placed.

Ralph lived in continual fear. He suffered from stomach and muscular problems, for he had no concept of what it meant to relax. He worried that if he relaxed, he would drop his guard and therefore be vulnerable to attack. He worried that someone would take advantage of him and as a result he would be damaged irreparably. He was worried that he was his father.

Ralph did not want to go through his father's life-defining experience of losing his job, savings, and house. This experience was traumatic enough, but the way his parents handled it made it exponentially worse. They simply refused to discuss it. Ralph's father acted as though nothing had changed. Even as the family wondered where their next meal was coming from, Dad continued to position himself as a captain of industry and a legendary financial success. This high-intensity denial was fueled and exacerbated by his father's increased drinking. Ralph's family had also gone into abject denial about his father's alcoholism. It was only years later that Ralph realized his father had been a functional alcoholic long before the downfall. In fact, he remembered his father drinking highballs as soon as he came home from work.

Ralph wondered why his parents had even bothered to have children since they did not spend time with them or take the effort to nurture them. When Ralph was in his forties, his father was dying of cancer. Ralph decided that he would visit his father daily in order to provide him emotional support. He also desperately wanted his father to express his feelings as he now faced the end of his life, to talk about the tragedy that had caused him to lose everything. Ralph attempted every strategy he could imagine to facilitate this. Day after day he sat and talked with his father, but the older man remained a master of denial. He would not even mention the fact that he was dying or that he had any illness at all.

Ralph was uncertain as to how he should deal with his father's reluctance to share his feelings. He didn't want to play the denial game any longer, but he had no support from other family members. Ralph ached to be close to his father, and he was hungry for a physical embrace. Sadly, though, Ralph's dream of building an emotional bridge between himself and his dad never came true. One winter morning he received word from his mother that his dad had died in his sleep.

Ralph felt like he had fallen off a cliff. He was profoundly frightened as he realized that not only would he not get the answers that he needed from his father, but he would also never have the opportunity to get emotionally close to him. Ralph felt that now he would never know if his father loved him because his dad had never uttered the words to tell him so. Ralph's dad had never in any way praised or even hugged his son.

Ralph learned in therapy that he had not accepted the fact that his father had died. Ralph in all his attempts to achieve perfection was still trying to gain approval from his father. He could not come to terms with the reality that he would never get his father's love.

Ralph's sense of failure in the eyes of his father caused him to become agitated, anxious, and depressed. Since it is humanly impossible to be perfect, Ralph visited these debilitating emotional states on a daily basis. His extremely unrealistic expectations fed his need to control every aspect of his life and the lives of those around him. He had to know what would happen when he died; belief or faith was not enough. He had to know that his kids would do well in college before they were even accepted into a university. He worried constantly that his wife's diabetes would make her very sick and kill her, and he found himself in prolonged states of panic because he believed that his life would be over if hers ended. Catastrophe seemed inevitable on every level.

Although he attended psychotherapy sessions regularly for a year, out of shame Ralph did not reveal the intensity of his anxiety and depression. He was humiliated that he could not live up to his own expectations of perfection. Ralph had never had a close relationship with his father, but he'd always wanted one. Since his father had shared nothing of his inner world, Ralph had shaped his own mythology about how the way his father's mind worked. The myth held that his father was perfect both in his financial vision and in its execution; that whatever moneymaking plan he conceived was successfully realized. This myth was not only untrue; it was diametrically opposed to reality.

Ralph, like many people immersed in fear, did not believe there was a different way to deal with his anxiety. He certainly did not believe that the answers to his angst resided inside him. Only when he began to change his belief system about the possibility of healing could he discover that the answers resided in his heart. Ralph reached a crossroads in his life: He could continue to live in his chaotic, nightmarish fashion, or he could find an alternative. As he became sick and tired of going down the same fear-based, unsatisfying, dead-ending path his life had taken, he became more acutely aware that his disruptive behavior was pushing away those closest to him.

Ralph began to realize that he was angry at his father and that he had repressed this anger for many years. Slowly he came to accept that his dad was like all of us, flawed. He was eventually able to face the sad fact that his father had never been there for him and had never taught him how to use his own internal resources. Ralph recognized that he couldn't ever meet his father and repair their relationship, but he could learn to heal himself.

He made a concerted effort to be less protective of his children and less possessive of his wife. Instead of placing a tremendous amount of pressure on her by demanding her attendance at all times, Ralph learned to be supportive of her desire to control her diabetes. One indication that Ralph was no longer in denial of his angst was that he opened himself up to discussion of his worries and fears in a sincere manner. Ralph reached another milestone when he accepted that utilizing anti-anxiety medication was a helpful tool during this crisis.

None of these transformations would have been effective without Ralph's bold determination to improve the quality of his life. His journey continues.

Elaine G., the thirty-eight-year-old woman from New Orleans introduced in chapter 2, also had a parent problem. Her mother was a prominent executive whose extensive travel kept her away from home much of the time, so Elaine was essentially raised by nannies. Her mother had married twice. Elaine's father had died when she was only seven years old, and she does not remember that he paid much attention to her. Her mother's second husband didn't work at all, but he had any number of get-rich-quick schemes that never panned out. As he had no money of his own, he had to depend upon his wife for the money to fund his projects, which she continued to provide, even though they invariably failed.

Elaine describes her mother as being demanding and unaffectionate. While she expected Elaine to win all of the art contests she regularly entered and to do well academically, her mother did not seem to care if Elaine was actually happy or not. Elaine always felt that her mother saw her more as an object than as her daughter.

Elaine's mother did not encourage her to develop friendships or enjoy spontaneous fun. The combination of Elaine's mother rarely being home with her inability to nurture Elaine when she was, prevented the development of a healthy mother-child bond. Therefore, Elaine was closer to her favorite nanny, Beth, who was the complete antithesis of her mom. If Beth noticed that Elaine was fearful for any reason, she would comfort her and not allow Elaine to be by herself. As a result of the nanny's continual intervention, Elaine never learned how to soothe herself when she was fearful. Her fears eventually escalated into full-blown panic attacks.

Beth essentially performed the maternal functions Elaine's mother did not. And Beth's values differed substantially from those of Elaine's mother; as focused as Elaine's mother was on money and status, Beth focused on close relationships and genuineness. Elaine realized that she was constantly moving internally from the world of her mother to the world of Beth.

When I first saw Elaine, her marriage at age twenty-three to Craig, a very wealthy man, had recently ended after fifteen years. Elaine had been elated to marry someone of Craig's station. Not only was he rich, but he had the premium status and aura of invincibility associated with the society's cream of the crop. Elaine felt protected by him; he gave her the sense of family she'd never had before. She also loved the charity benefits and the cocktail parties they attended regularly.

Gradually, though, Craig's affection toward Elaine diminished. He was spending more and more time away from home, and he became very distant. He stopped being sexual with her. Yet he never explained why he was pushing her out of his life.

Instead he denied that anything was wrong, and this exacerbated Elaine's sense of loneliness. In time, Elaine realized she was very unhappy in her marriage and that Craig was not a loving person. Elaine interpreted his lack of any affection as rejection. One day she walked out of the marriage.

And out of a life. Elaine was shocked when her so-called friends from charity benefits no longer spoke to her when she encountered them. At the same time, the invitations to high-profile social events stopped arriving. As her world began to crumble, Elaine felt overwhelmed with sadness at the loss of her marriage. She felt like a failure.

Elaine is a very articulate, vivacious person. She had spent considerable time formulating the reasons why she was seeking therapy. During our first session, she talked about the panic attacks that had begun in childhood and continued to this point in her life. She wanted to understand what these panic attacks were about; she wanted to know how she could end them for good. Afraid of being alone, Elaine had a daily schedule that assured that she'd not be by herself for any length of time. Her fear had become a crippling emotional disability, and she was filled with shame to even think about it.

Her mother was now elderly and quite ill. While Elaine was worried and concerned that her mother didn't have much time left on earth, at the same time she was filled with mixed emotions. Mostly she was very angry with her mother for not being around when she was growing up. She wondered if it would be possible for her to work through these issues with her mom; she wondered if she even wanted to do so.

Elaine described her panic-attack symptoms: an elevated heart rate, sweating, an uncomfortable feeling of fear filling her body, then feeling that the panic state would last forever, and the space she was in was getting gradually smaller, uncertainty about what to do to calm herself, hyperventilating. Her panic attacks begin when no one else is apparently present, either at home or away from home, as in a dead quiet neighborhood. The panic can be triggered when she is driving and suddenly notices that she's alone—nobody else appears to be around. At that point, in a state of panic, she drives around in search of other people. Once she sees another person, or even another moving vehicle, her symptoms ease considerably. She says that her panic attacks are caused by the irrational feeling that everyone on earth has left and that everyone has abandoned her.

Elaine's panic attacks are not only exhausting experiences; they also tend to diminish her self-esteem and confidence. Because Elaine believes that she has to have a relationship with a man in order to feel safe, she chooses men who will be at her beck and call. These relationships inevitability prove to be unfulfilling because the connection with her partner centers entirely on her need never to be alone. While these men tend to make themselves present whenever she requests, they don't satisfy her intellectual, professional, or creative needs. They diminish rather than enhance Elaine's self.

The panic attacks originated in Elaine's childhood. Her parents were totally uninvolved in the emotional development of their daughter. Even though they knew that Elaine became nervous at the prospect of being alone, they did nothing to allay her fears. Instead, they passed on their parental responsibilities to Elaine's nannies.

All children experience fear in their young lives; indeed, learning that being afraid is normal is a significant milestone in child development. Parents involved in the emotional growth of their children reassure them that monsters won't be breaking down their doors and teach them to focus on something else if they become scared. They encourage their kids to share feelings of dread. In this way parents can teach their kids to distinguish between an irrational fear and a real one. For instance, while explaining that monsters don't exist, they might also point out that the neighborhood bully is someone to avoid; they might even enroll the child in a self-defense class. If a child leaves his room in the middle of the night because he is scared to be alone, the right response for parents is to soothe him and then ask him to return to his room. Realizing that his parents will not allow him stay in their room, the child will try to calm himself, perhaps by reading and thinking about his favorite superhero. He will look inside himself for ways to face fear.

Elaine's parents did nothing of the sort to help her face and diminish her fears. While her parents were neglectful, Elaine's nanny was emotionally intrusive; she may have encouraged little Elaine to be overly dependent on her.

Elaine's marriage collapsed gradually. Her first husband, Craig, was not willing to attend therapy sessions to work out their problems, and he became increasingly distant as time went on. Although she was the one to take the initial steps to end the marriage, three years after the divorce she still felt extremely traumatized. She had loved the social benefits of her marriage like the charity fundraising parties and the fashion shows. Her paintings were often displayed at these high-profile events, and for the first time she felt that she had a family, a husband and two glowing children, she could also show off. Though she was remarkably intelligent, process-oriented, and creative, Elaine nonetheless seemed to delight in the superficial duties that attended being the trophy wife of a wealthy man in the community.

Shortly after her marriage ended, Elaine began a relationship with another man. Tom was interested in going on vacations and having fun, and he was willing to be available whenever Elaine needed him. A computer programmer, Tom worked at several different companies in a few years' time. Elaine described him as being restless, unsure of what he wanted to do. Then he came to a professional halt; laid off from his job, he put forth little effort and no energy in securing a new position. Soon he was living off Elaine's money, and he became increasingly resentful that he was dependent on her for financial assistance. Elaine, in turn, became increasingly needy. She wanted Tom to be around her all the time. Meanwhile her panic attacks were occurring with more frequency and intensity. Elaine has come to realize that Tom is currently playing the role of codependent; he is in fact enabling her to remain immobile, paralyzed by fear.

It is not surprising that Elaine feels extremely vulnerable and dependent. While she has the benefit of many luxuries, financial freedom, intelligence, and leisure time, she feels like a prisoner. She feels guilty, too, for she believes it is an insult to God to have been given so many blessings without being able to enjoy them. It makes her feel like a "sinner" and an ingrate. She doesn't like the feelings. She desires to regain control of her destiny and start living the life she should be living.

Elaine is now committed to freeing herself from her fears. She forces herself to tolerate situations in which she is alone. While such occasions are rare and brief at the present time, this is a great and positive start.

Lucia is a forty-five-year-old woman from Los Angeles. She has been in therapy on several occasions to deal with the inordinate number of personal tragedies in her life. Nearly her entire family has died. Her mother died of cancer when Lucia was in her early twenties. Her father died of a heart attack when she was thirty-five. Her youngest brother died of a heroin overdose when she was in her teens. Her oldest sister died when Lucia was forty. Four years later her other sister died of a heart attack, and her oldest brother died of liver cancer when she was forty-five. These deaths have left her feeling raw, emotionally damaged, and confused.

Lucia describes her mother as having been distant and withdrawn, a woman who spent much of her time closed up in her room. In Lucia's view, her mother was depressed, alcoholic, and non-nurturing. She does not remember her mother ever praising her efforts or offering her any emotional support. Lucia did not feel that she could go to her mother if she was upset or curious or confused about the process of growing up. As she grew more aware, Lucia longed to free her mother from her misery, but she had no idea how to accomplish it. Her inability to fulfill this wish left Lucia feeling powerless and plagued her with guilt and remorse.

Lucia's father, a police officer on the streets of LA, identified strongly with his work and wasn't home very much. Lucia always felt that she was his favorite and that he loved her unconditionally. Still, he never seemed to be very involved in her life. He didn't encourage her to pursue her interests or even ask her what they were. He never looked at her report card and didn't seem to care if she was academically successful or not.

When Lucia was seven, one of her sisters pressed a pillow over her face in an effort to suffocate her, "If you weren't born," she shouted, "I would be getting the attention from Mom and Dad instead of you." Somehow, Lucia was able to force the pillow and her sister off her face and body. She remembers her sister crying when it was all over. Lucia saw no reason to inform her parents of her sister's attack, simply because they wouldn't want to hear about it. Experience had already taught Lucia that the only person she could count on was herself. She'd learned not to reach out to others.

Lucia's parents did not teach their daughter how to deal with death. It, like other uncomfortable topics, was taboo for discussion. This unwritten family rule of not discussing any topic that was potentially disturbing played a major role in Lucia's life. When she felt the onset of sadness for her family's losses, she tried to push her feelings aside as she felt they were inappropriate. She'd learned that sadness, for instance, was an emotion not to be expressed; for her parents met her tears with only indifference or anger.

Anger, however, was an acceptable and indeed encouraged emotion. It was OK to yell and scream at each other; it was all right even to become physically violent with each other. Yet these expressions of rage led to nothing constructive. Experiences were not processed, emotions were not released, nothing was resolved.

It is a common belief that the physical or verbal expression of anger will facilitate the release of pent-up hostility. Supposedly, one feels calmness afterward, and a sense of inner peace. Actually, this calmness is momentary. The "release" that is experienced does not resolve the issues that created the anger in the first place. The physical act of hitting someone or breaking something provides the same type of relief as finally finding a bathroom when you really have to go. Screaming obscenities at someone or deeply demeaning a person's character provides an adrenaline rush much like the kick when ingesting cocaine or speed. Again, though, the high is temporary. This acted-out rage, like a drug rush, fades quickly and is replaced with emptiness, guilt, and confusion.

Lucia's family members fought constantly over trivial and serious matters alike. She would yell at her brothers and sisters, and they would berate her in kind. Their fighting did not solve any problems, but it did provide a quick outlet of emotional expression that also distracted them from their depressive mother's alcoholism and their younger brother's drug addiction.

Lucia's younger brother had drug problems throughout most

of his adolescence. If her father was largely uninvolved during this long crisis, her mother enabled him. She did not set limits on him, did not push him to take responsibility for his life. She enabled him by ignoring and denying his drug usage. She also encouraged Lucia to help her brother by being kind to him. The message that Lucia got from her mother was that she was responsible for her brother's well-being. As a result, Lucia, like her mother, participated in her brother's drug addiction. Lucia's personality came to be defined by her codependence.

Lucia's codependent behavior prompted her to place everyone's needs before her own. Because she felt that the well-being of those closest to her was her ultimate duty, she felt constantly disappointed as she was certain to fail in these endeavors. Outside the family home she would unconsciously seek out intimate relationships and friendships with people who were deeply wounded emotionally. Her behavior assumed a pattern: Lucia would attempt to provide moral support, finances, transportation, and love to jobless people who wouldn't look for work; to alcoholics and drug addicts who refused to seek rehab; to depressed and anxious folks who shunned the idea of therapy; and to physically ill folks who would skip doctor appointments. As Lucia saw it, her job was to heal other people's wounds. Despite her intelligence and insightfulness, Lucia could not see that her friends or lovers made little or no effort to heal themselves. Furthermore, Lucia's fixation with enabling others prevented her from attending to her own needs, a common side effect of being overly codependent. Indeed, Lucia did not think about her own educational, emotional, or professional desires; she would feel guilty and put them aside.

When one loved one after another died with little duration between losses, Lucia had trouble grieving because she had never learned how. The added dimension of her enabling behavior made her feel, too, that she hadn't done enough to save her family members from dying. In addition, she felt survivor's guilt: Why she was the only member of her family left alive?

How this combination of issues affected Lucia is best illustrated by her relationship with her sister Silvia, the sister who attempted to suffocate Lucia when she was a child. Silvia was always sickly and never had a job. Her father provided for her until his death, at which point she became eligible for social security because she was legally disabled. Silvia suffered extreme depression and she was deeply resentful of Lucia. Silvia believed that once her younger sister came into the world, her parents ceased paying attention to her; and she held on to this belief her entire life. She had few interests other than junk food and television.

However much Lucia found her sister to be demanding and inconsiderate, Silvia had programmed her to believe that it was Lucia's responsibility to drop whatever she was doing to come to her older sister's aid. Silvia had arthritis, among other painful health problems, but she was a very noncompliant patient. She was inconsistent in taking her medicine, she didn't eat healthy foods, and she refused to exercise. She complained to Lucia about her plight, but she made no effort at self-care. All of this increased Lucia's sense of guilt. She would get stomach aches from wondering what she needed to do in order to make Silvia happy. It didn't dawn on her until much later that Silvia was responsible for her own joy.

The revelation came to Lucia shortly before Silvia's death. Silvia had developed heart problems, and Lucia was visiting her daily, a tedious routine as Lucia had already put in a ten-hour workday. She gradually realized that no matter what comfort, support, or guidance she delivered to her older sister, nothing helped. Silvia continued to telegraph Lucia the message that Lucia's very existence was the reason she was so miserable. She also made it quite clear that Lucia owed her for the transfer of their parents' attention after she was born. Silvia held on to this resentment for more than forty years. Finally Lucia realized that this "debt" could never be repaid because it was impossible to pay for a crime she didn't commit. She realized that Silvia should have confronted her parents with her resentment rather than acting it out in her relationship with Lucia.

One day Silvia called Lucia at work and reached her voice mail because she was in a meeting. Lucia was tired of trying to placate her sister and felt that it was time for her to take some responsibility for herself, so she didn't call her back as soon as she got the message. That evening, Silvia ended up in the hospital with heart problems. The doctors wanted her to stay a few days to run tests, but she left against medical advice. Silvia died of a heart attack a few days later.

At this point Lucia had mixed feelings about her sister's death. She felt guilty that she wasn't there for her at the end of her life, but she was angry that Silvia's unwillingness to take care of herself had caused her to lose her life prematurely at age fifty-three. Lucia was sad, too, because her sister had missed all the opportunities life could offer—she'd never had a primary relationship, had few friends, never had a career, and never gone to college.

As she began to examine her own life, Lucia realized that she had developed her enabling personality through her interaction with her dysfunctional family. She began to gain confidence and understand the concept of personal boundaries. She learned to concentrate on herself without feeling selfish. She became able to tolerate the mixed feelings that she had for her sister. Finally, she was no longer afraid to face the sad, angry, and confusing feelings she had about all the deaths in her family.

Camille P. is a fifty-year-old woman who lives in Southern California. Her mother was Caucasian and her father Filipino. She sought out therapy several years ago, soon after her husband died. She is now a single mother raising three children. She has some family and friends in the area, but both her parents died years ago. She is used to taking care of herself and not reaching out for support.

Camille's childhood was constantly in a state of upheaval. Her mother suffered schizophrenia, a mental disorder that plagued her with visual and auditory hallucinations; unfortunately it was diagnosed only after her death. Camille describes her mother's behavior as erratic; when she became angry, she also became physically and emotionally abusive and would fly into uncontrollable rages during which she'd break glassware, cry, and scream aspersions she said she heard people saying about her. Her father was an alcoholic whose drinking was out of control. He spent much of his time away from the home; in fact, he had another residence in a town forty miles away where he was employed as a cook. Camille remembers that her father was around so infrequently that when he was, he kept mostly to himself in the kitchen, drinking. Camille learned early to stay away from both her parents as much as possible, since her mother's rage was often directed at Camille and her father, who got belligerent when drunk, frequently becoming physically and emotionally abusive to her.

Camille grew up in a two-story home in which the primary living area was upstairs. On the first level were the garage and an extra room quite removed from the rest of the home. When Camille was seven years old, her mother decided that her daughter should move into the spare room near the basement. The room was cold and remote, with wall-to-wall windows on three sides of the room. The windows had no curtains, and a bare light bulb blared from the overhead fixture. They put a bed into the room, and Camille moved into this space in the hope that she could escape her parents' abuse. She spent much of her time reading or drawing but all the while listening for her mother's call, which she could hear from the heater vent. The door to the room had a small window through which Camille could see the front door to the house at the end of a long straight hallway.

Camille was ten years old on what she describes as an unusual Sunday, in that her father was home; this wasn't his normal schedule. It was late in the evening and she was upstairs when she heard her mother crying. At about 11:00 p.m., she went down to her bedroom. In what seemed like only minutes she heard a loud explosion come from upstairs. She looked out the window of her room and down the long hallway but saw nothing. She opened her door and heard her brother's voice calling 911 and saying that someone had been shot. Their mother always kept a loaded pistol by her bedside, and in that moment Camille could only conclude that either her mother or father had been shot. Frightened, in a state of panic, Camille stepped out of her room and started to walk down the long hallway that would take her upstairs. She was halfway down the hall when her brother appeared and told her to go back to her room until someone came and got her. Her brother would not tell her what had happened. Camille did what she was told but watched through the window of her bedroom door. She remembers the police and fire department coming into the house through the front door and, sometime later, a gurney with a body entirely covered up being wheeled away. Camille waited up all night for someone to come and get her, but no one ever came. She sat wondering who had died, her mother or her father. Apparently no one was concerned that she was alone in the room downstairs. The next morning was a school day, so a tentative Camille dressed and went upstairs. It was immediately evident that her mother was gone, as Camille's father met her at the top of the stairs. He told her to come with him into her mother's bedroom, and then led her to the spot where her mother had shot and killed herself. There was a massive amount of blood on the carpet; Camille remembers just staring at it, transfixed. Then her father said, "Your mother is dead. Do you want to go to school?" In shock, Camille said yes, she wanted to go to school. Soon after, Camille's two older sisters arrived at the house and her father also took them into the room. Her sisters decided Camille should not go to school. She spent the rest of her day with her sisters making the funeral arrangements. When the three of them arrived back at home, all of their mother's clothes and personal items were gone. So were Camille's pets, a dog and a rabbit. That everything belonging to her mother had been removed was never questioned. No one spoke about it or even asked what happened. For years the entire incident remained undiscussed.

Her father responded by moving the family, which now consisted of Camille and her older brother, to another house. There they were essentially left to fend for themselves, as their father was not around during much of the week. Whatever else he was doing, he was also looking for a wife, often bringing different women around to meet her and her brother. Not more than six months after her mother's death, her father remarried and started a new life; it did not include Camille or her brother. Camille never lived with her father again.

Now living with one of her sisters, Camille began to have problems with sore throats. They became so frequent that a tonsillectomy was performed. Because Camille had been staying with her sister for a few months prior to the surgery, she expected to go from the hospital to her sister's house. Instead, she was picked up at the hospital and taken to the "home" that her father had rented for her and her brother to live in on their own.

Camille's father had the carpet removed from the room where her mother had committed suicide and had it installed in the new house, in what was Camille's bedroom. Camille remembers being horrified on seeing her mother's bloodstains on the carpet. She couldn't imagine why her father had chosen to do this. Was he oblivious to the stains? Was he interested only in saving the money that a new carpet would cost? Did he simply not care how his children might react to this traumatic reminder of the last day of their mother's life?

Three years older than she, Camille's brother was physically abusive to her; beat up on her on a regular basis. Camille didn't ask her father for help because she felt that he didn't really care what happened to her. Since she could not rely on family for anything, she learned to trust her own mind to figure out how to survive. She completed her schoolwork with no one's assistance. She found work as a teenager so that she'd have her own money, and as soon as she was old enough, she enrolled in a school-sponsored work program. She moved out of her house when she was seventeen and worked full-time to financially support herself. Many times she had to work two jobs just to survive.

At the time she began therapy, Camille was working as an executive in a high-profile computer software company. She loved her job and the financial rewards that came with it. She became so consumed with her work that she was able to temporarily disconnect from the grief she experienced when her husband died.

Camille, however, did deeply feel her children's pain after their father's death and was willing to do virtually anything to buffer their loss. She assumed their household chores; she allowed them to be disrespectful without any meaningful consequences; she did not discipline them when they disregarded the rules and did poorly in school, and she did not set limits. This is actually a common reaction. The loss of a family member or close relative prompts parents often to feel so sorry for their children that they literally let them get away with anything. The parent, too, may often be so caught up in working through her own grief that she does not have the energy to set proper limits and provide guidance and direction.

Camille and her children continued this way of living for years. The children had difficult teenage years and have had problems functioning as young adults, what with their anger management issues and lack of direction.

Since her husband's death, Camille has had several relationships with men. They all tend to share the same characteristics: an unpredictable temper; substance abuse problems; emotional unavailability; a seemingly caring, thoughtful nature at the beginning of the relationship and an increasingly harsh attitude toward Camille over time. Camille has trouble ending these relationships. Even in the face of obvious signs that the relationship is not working, she endures continual abuse long before she does anything about it. Some of these men went out of control under the influence of alcohol and became physically and verbally abusive.

Camille desires an intimate relationship, but she chooses men who she finds offputting at times. When she confronts these men regarding their insensitive actions, she inevitably wins any ensuing argument. While significant men in her life almost invariably prove to be unchallenging on an intellectual level, they are challenging on an emotional one. Camille claims to be interested in what makes them "tick." Unconsciously she hopes to mold them into her fantasy expectations; an impossible hope, so therefore it fails. Camille is thus constantly disappointed. She is aware that she herself is partially responsible for her disappointment in that.

She is frightened of allowing herself to get too close to a man, but she doesn't know why.

Camille met all the requirements for super-employee. She was creative and thoughtful; she worked until the job got done. It was not unusual for her to work twelve-hour days. By immersing herself in work, she was able to escape from her personal problems.

Then she began to feel increasingly fatigued; she had little appetite. She was diagnosed with lupus. There is no known cure for lupus, which can be fatal, although it is possible to prolong life with steroids and other heavy-duty medications that can have severe side effects like weight gain, lethargy, rashes, difficulty concentrating, increased or decreased appetite, depression, anxiety, and abrupt mood swings.

Camille can no longer work and has applied for disability. Her insurance company has not gone out of its way to help her, and has in fact obstructed her every move to obtain assistance. Camille is still pursuing the complicated process of securing disability funding.

Nowadays, Camille doesn't know how she will feel when she wakes up in the morning. Some mornings she has a ton of energy and feels optimistic about the day to come. On other days, she is feverish with achy joints and a headache, and that makes her feel her situation is hopeless.

All of this has been devastating to her. However, Camille carefully looks at all the options available and makes plans based on those options. Those options are: ignoring the disability insurance process and trying to work; doing as much research as possible on disability insurance; finding the funds to hire a disability insurance advocate; or just give up. She is a survivor, so she won't give up. Indeed, many child-abuse victims have incredible survival skills. Without parental encouragement and community support, they find the strength within themselves to not only survive, but also to succeed.

Even though her health and finances are in crisis, Camille is determined to resolve her problems with primary relationships. She now understands that having relationships with men who are unaware of her emotional wounds gives her a sense of control that she doesn't possess in any other facets of her life. One man with whom she was recently involved was extremely inconsiderate and self-absorbed, but Camille had no inhibitions about confronting him on his latest selfish act. He was more concerned about minor car engine trouble than her debilitating illness. She gave him a detailed, scathing analysis of his behavior without pulling any punches. In doing so, she gained a sense of power that distracted her from her tribulations.

Camille, amazingly enough, is not only focused on her own survival. She is also seeking peace of mind and happiness. She has come to realize that her relationships with these deeply emotionally wounded men are connected to her unhappy relationship with her father. Her father was emotionally distant, and Camille recalls her desire to feel loved by him. She believed that if she could ease his pain and stop his drinking, he would finally shower her with affection. She is now aware that she has continued to repeat this pattern with all the other significant men in her life, and she is fighting for solutions. To some degree Camille was able to attain some intellectual clarity about her relationship with her father when he became ill with cancer and she was caring for him after his surgery. After decades of emotional distance from her father, she began to feel close to him for the first time. She tried very hard to understand him so that she could better understand herself and move forward in her own life.

Sarah W., a forty-three-year-old woman, one day realized that she had been depressed and anxious most of her life. She was spending an extraordinary amount of time sleeping, and when she was awake she felt hopeless, lethargic, and out of control. She worried constantly about the well-being of others and forecast the worst possible outcome for nearly whatever situation her family or friends might find themselves in.

Sarah's parents were working poor folks who lived in a small town in Vermont. Her father worked in a factory while her mother took care of Sarah, her two brothers, and her one sister. Sarah left home as soon as she could, at age eighteen, and moved to Los Angeles. There she met a banking industry executive, a man on his way up, whom she saw as a means to escape poverty. She had two children with him, boys, one year apart. It soon became apparent, though, that her husband was a self-absorbed alcoholic oblivious to anyone's concerns but his own. Sarah spent much of her time trying to compensate for the lack of love and affection the children received from their father. As they grew older, Sarah continued to try to protect them from the pain as well as the normal anguishes all children experience outside the home.

Sarah had grown up in a small Vermont town where nearly everyone was poor. It was as if the Great Depression had never ended. For thirty years, her father worked in the same factory where he never received a promotion and never complained. Her father believed that whatever job you had, whatever home you lived in, whatever car you drove, whatever school your children went to, all was what it was supposed to be and no one had the right to question it. He seemed genuinely to be convinced that a person had no right to aspire to anything beyond his or her current station in life. Therefore, when Sarah talked to her father about going to college, he ridiculed her: Girls didn't go to college, he said; they stayed home, made babies, and took care of their men.

There was a distinct lack of joy in the household. Every day you just got up, went to work, came home, had a couple of beers, and went to bed, and you kept doing this until the day you died. The beers were a problem for Sarah's father; he consumed a lot more than a couple every day. Sarah doesn't remember her father being a mean drunk; what sticks out the most in her memory of him is that she felt reduced by him to the point of invisibility. To him, girls were inferior to boys. So her brothers had several sets of clothes while she had to make do with only one dress. Neither her mother nor father complimented her on her good grades. If anything, they saw her high academic performance as a threat to the natural order of the household.

Her mother's job was to enable her husband to maintain his daily routine by keeping a clean house, and buying groceries and alcohol. Sarah never felt that her mother even thought to protect her, and one particularly traumatic event underscored that belief. One day, when Sarah was about eight years old, her parents left her in the care of an uncle. Sarah remembers the uncle chasing her around his house and eventually fondling her. Terrified and traumatized by this event, she reported it to her mother, only to be told: "That didn't really happen. Why are you angry at your uncle? He is so good to you."

Sarah's mother was the queen of denial. She gave the incident of her daughter's sexual abuse incident no credence. She would dismiss without listening the possibility that her husband might be an alcoholic. Her attitude left Sarah feeling unsafe and unheard.

When Sarah's children became teenagers, she started psychotherapy. She was depressed, she was experiencing panic attacks. Her depression had gotten so bad that she'd seriously considered ending her life. Several nights a week she was polishing off a bottle of wine by herself. She could no longer tolerate her husband's rage at her and the children. He had become increasingly abusive over the years, though he never acknowledged that his behavior was anything but normal. He could not empathize with Sarah, would not ever think to try, and discounted her complaints, just as her father did years earlier.

Sarah reached the tipping point when her husband's abuse of her and neglect of the children became intolerable. She filed for divorce—a move that shocked and appalled her husband. The divorce was fraught with hostility. Sarah's husband refused to move out of the house until long after the divorce was final, and by then he began to have health problems related to aging, drinking, and the lack of self-care. He finally moved into a condo several miles away, but he insisted on celebrating holidays with Sarah and her children. He also insisted that Sarah drive him to his doctor appointments, and Sarah complied.

In the early stages of their divorce, Sarah heeded his demands because she felt responsible for him. Forever, it seemed, she had always felt that she was responsible for the well-being of those closest to her; she'd focused every moment of her days on the effort. Finally, though, she realized that this goal was unattainable. Not only were her family members difficult to please, it was impossible for her to clear the obstacles that were making them miserable. Only they could do that for themselves.

While fighting against the unexpressed emotional pain that her husband was experiencing, Sarah neglected her own needs, although she barely recognized that she herself had needs, let alone what they were. She didn't know, either, why her husband was so miserable, but she felt it was her job to uplift him. That he also denied he had any problems made it all the more difficult to connect with him.

Sarah began to realize, in therapy, that her relationship with her husband was similar to the one her mother had maintained with her father. Certainly there were similarities between her father and her husband. They were both emotionally unavailable alcoholics who believed that women were inferior to men. They were both self-involved, mean-spirited men who treated Sarah as if she was part of the dinette set. We tend to be attracted to partners who share personality traits with our parents. While we don't purposely choose people with our parents' qualities for lovers, it happens nonetheless on an unconscious level. Often our attraction to others lies in personality characteristics we find familiar because they were models for us when we were growing up. We initially feel comfortable with this familiarity as being safe and we know how to operate within it; it allows us to conform to long-established patterns from our childhood. Such partnership is also an unconscious effort to understand what went wrong in our relationships with our mother and father.

After the divorce, Sarah began having panic attacks with symptoms that included heart palpitations, sweating, feeling disoriented, and hyperventilating. They forced her to consider what exactly she was worried about. For one thing, she needed to find an occupation that would support her. For another, she needed to decide where she wanted to live and if she wanted her now-adult children to live with her. She realized she had no sense of identity apart from that of someone who took care of others. Perhaps this was the most frightening aspect of her new life. She was both excited and fearful at the prospect of the future.

During one of our sessions, Sarah had a panic attack in the midst of talking about her concerns. She didn't know how to get out of this state; she was breathing laboriously and in obvious discomfort. So I asked her, "Do you like the singer-songwriter Joan Armatrading?" She smiled, and we proceeded to talk about Armatrading's music and concerts for the next five minutes. Sarah soon realized that she was no longer having a panic attack. She had learned the technique of healthy distraction. Eventually, she understood that she could face important issues one at a time.

Sarah had wanted to be an interior decorator ever since she was a little girl. She finally realized this dream when she opened up her own business. She also decided to move out of the area, and she no longer returned her ex-husband's calls. She developed new friendships. She stopped abusing alcohol. Having faced the trauma of her uncle's sexual abuse, she recognizes that it had a profoundly negative effect on her self-esteem and sense of safety. She encourages her children to be independent, and they now live in places of their own. Sarah lets them know that she is available for support and problem-solving discussion, but she refuses to enable them. She has developed her own boundaries and has an internal awareness of the appropriate separation between herself and others. She has discovered an inner world, and she is tasting happiness.

Joan H. is a twenty-nine-year-old woman who grew up and lives in San Diego, California. She had excelled in theater ever since she was a little girl and actually obtained a college scholarship based on her acting abilities.

On the surface, Joan appeared to be a happy, well-adjusted kid who loved every sunny moment of her life. She was popular in school and participated in many community activities. She had a wonderful reputation with teachers because of her hard work in and out of the classroom, her dedication to theater, and her unfailing reliability. None of her friends or the teachers she was close to was aware of the angst she was experiencing on a daily basis.

Joan's father was also an actor; however, he was not as talented as his daughter was, and he had difficulty accepting that fact. He was constantly putting her down and attacking her character. Joan describes him as being very critical of her on a daily basis. His criticism was both overt and subtle. If she scored a B instead of an A on a test, he would call her stupid and contend that she would never make it in the world. When she received raves for her theatrical performances, he would disguise his contempt for her with "constructive criticism."

Furthermore, Joan's father seemed to hate every aspect of his own life. He didn't like his management job because it was too boring, he despised his wife and mostly ignored her, and he was resentful that he had to provide a place to live for his directionless younger brother.

This brother, Joan's uncle, was literally torturing Joan almost every day. He would tie her up and beat her until she was black and blue, but with the bruises hidden under her clothes, Joan was able to conceal her shame at school and the community. Her uncle threatened to rape her and he did fondle her at times. Joan complained to her parents about the physical abuse, but she kept the sexual abuse a secret. Regardless, her parents did nothing. Her father simply didn't believe her; he said she was making up stories in order to get attention. Her mother responded to Joan's pleas that she do something to halt the uncle's aggression by asking him to stop hurting Joan. Her uncle would give her mother assurances, then resume the abuse the next day.

Joan felt unsafe in her own home, and because of her lack of security she was afraid to reveal her uncle's abuse either to peers or to adults she looked up to. She feared her uncle's retaliation.

Joan learned to bottle up her sadness and anger over her uncle's hurtful behavior. When one denies their angry and sad feelings, however, they don't just disappear. They exhibit themselves in physical discomforts like muscle pain, headaches, and stomach aches.

Joan acted out indirectly. As she grew into adolescence, her rage poured out of her stressed soul more and more. She began having angry outbursts at school if she felt she'd been disrespected by a classmate. She would threaten to physically harm anyone who she thought had hurt or betrayed her. None of the school personnel could get a handle on what was troubling Joan. Although she continued to excel academically and in theater, it was clear to all those who knew her well that she was deeply troubled about something.

Joan went to college in New Jersey, where her life went into a downward spiral. She was eighteen; she was on her own for the first time. At last now he was now free from her father's insults and her uncle's terrorism. She might have been relieved, but Joan didn't respond that way. She deadened her emotions; she succumbed to the anesthetizing effects of marijuana and alcohol. She used them to combat her intense loneliness during her first semester at college. She found her homework to be difficult and her classes to be boring and irrelevant. She had a series of boyfriends who she felt were interested less in her than they were in sex. She unable to find a professor who could mentor her or a teacher she could confide in. She felt lost.

Joan knew that she was deep in the land of self-destruction

when she found herself missing drama classes and rehearsals. She ended her first semester with an F every class. Her poor performance allowed her father to confirm his lack of faith in her. Her mother just shook her head and offered no comfort. Joan dropped out of college realizing that she needed help; she began treatment and worked hard to end her abuse of pot and alcohol. She took a job as a factory worker and found an apartment. She developed confidence and a sense of independence. She was living alone, three thousand miles away from her parents and uncle. She'd started to make new friends. She was managing to stay clean and sober.

Several years later Joan married a pilot for a major airline. She was now working in community theater where she taught children's drama. She considered it her dream job, and she was generally quite content and pleased with her life. But past issues suddenly bolted into the present.

In the beginning of their marriage, Joan's husband had a flight schedule that allowed him to be home on most days. During their third year together, though, this arrangement changed and he was away from home a week at a time every other week. Increasingly, loneliness dominated Joan's world. She felt so alone the week that her husband was gone that she would cry herself to sleep. Then she met a man at work, and they began a passionate affair.

This man told Joan about his terrible childhood; his father who slapped him across the face for the sport of it and his mother who literally attempted to poison him. Joan found his personal history to be as intoxicating to her as her heavy drinking and drug experiences had been. She became addicted to him and needed to know where he was every minute of the day. He became her crusade; she set out to fix what was broken inside him. She bought him music CDs, wrote him poetry, and brought him his favorite dessert in order to lift his spirits. But she had undertaken a thankless and unfulfilling task; for no matter what she did, she could never get him out of his doldrums.

Still, rescuing him remained Joan's number one priority. The more unresponsive he seemed to be to her efforts to save him, the more determined she became. His rejection further fueled her rescue mission. Joan got so caught up in the process that she was blind to what was really going on. It didn't dawn on her that she couldn't save him, that it was his job to deal with his own misery. Yet, she knew her relationship with him was wrong for any number of other reasons and she began searching for ways to end it. She sought out therapy for the second time in her life. She needed to understand how she had fallen into this self-destructive mess and wanted to address what was driving her to sabotage her marriage and her well-being.

She came to realize that since childhood she'd felt that no one was ever there for her when she needed them. Her father lashed out in his hatred toward her, her uncle controlled her through physical and sexual torture, and her mother pretended nothing awful was really happening. No one listened to her; she had no voice. Joan learned, too, that she did not really know how to be close with a partner. She perceived rescuing as a means to achieving intimacy. She began to understand what her attempt to "save" was all about. Joan believed that if she saved this man from his own demons, he would suddenly appreciate her and give her the love that she had never received from her parents.

Joan is an intelligent, witty, energetic woman whose new insight into herself is allowing her to slowly let go of a dysfunctional relationship. She still sees this man, although they stopped being sexual months ago. And she still experiences pain when he disappoints her, but each of their encounters now has the effect of clarifying further one fact: that this relationship has to end completely. She reports that her relationship with her husband is improving. She is enjoying her time with him and opening up to him more than she had previously. She is also working on understanding what role the physical and sexual abuse in her childhood and adolescence has had on her life. She is brave and determined. She is working it out.

William C. is a thirty-five-year-old man who originally sought therapy three years ago because he was in crisis. His marriage was in trouble; his professional life was in danger of collapsing. He was having physical problems; in tremendous pain due to a motorcycle accident, he had become addicted to pain medication. And he wasn't suffering in silence. He'd involved all of his friends, family, and business associates in his daily drama.

William and his wife cared about each other deeply, but they didn't know how to meet each other's emotional needs. Their frequent verbal battles often escalated to property destruction and domestic violence. On several occasions the police and legal system had been involved, with William and his wife both facing domestic abuse charges. Their relationship was filled with chaos, personal attacks, and rejection. They took turns moving out of their house to stay with friends or family.

William talked to everyone about his problems. He lived in a small town in Florida, and all the townsfolk seemed to know his business. His day-to-day calamities were entertainment for the citizens. He would tell strangers and acquaintances alike the most intimate details of his life. He was desperate for their approval, and he believed that if he related his heartfelt woes to them, they would become friends for life. Instead, they avoided him. His friends and employees ended up either bailing out on him or manipulating him financially. William ended up feeling bitter, resentful, and hurt.

As a general contractor, William had developed a successful business. However, at times he personalized business discussions with clients and then felt victimized by them. He had a very difficult time accepting responsibility for his actions. While he would give lip service to being accountable, he really believed that everyone else was responsible for his tumultuous marriage, destructive friendships, and drug addiction.

William's motorcycle accident had severely injured his knee. The surgery kept him off his feet for more than two months. He was meanwhile in a great deal of pain, which led to his addiction to Vicodin and other painkillers. Vicodin relaxes the body and mind to the point that one can feel euphoric. William experienced this sense of euphoria; but to attain it, as his tolerance to the drug gradually grew, he required a steadily increased dosage. When he found that the quantity prescribed by his physician failed to meet his needs, he began ordering the drug on the Internet. He recalls being so fixated on the drug that he learned the UPS truck's daily routes so he could intercept the package rather than wait for it to arrive at his home.

One of the many side effects of Vicodin is increased agitation, which made William only more disrespectful toward his wife. However justifiable may have been his reasons to be angry with her, he expressed his anger inappropriately. He would scream at her for hours, all the while demeaning her character and assaulting her with his words. He was constantly enraged at her, yet at the same time he was dependent on her and he resented it. Adept in financial matters, she handled the company's books. She cooked, she cleaned, tasks William hardly cared to undertake, and she was there for him when he required extra assistance after his knee injury. He knew, but would not admit even to himself, that she was the only person in the world he could really count on.

A knee injury like William's would be disruptive and disabling to anyone. For William it was catastrophic. He had been an all-county football player on his high school team enjoyed all of the perks afforded a star athlete. His parents demanded no chores or other responsibilities of him; they didn't expect him to excel academically. They did not teach him to be accountable. His mother, in particular, gave him the impression that he could do no wrong. She was reluctant to criticize or discipline him.

William's biological father left his mother and three small children when William was five years old. His father's departure was never explained, and William learned early on that this subject was taboo. His father also had substance abuse problems for much of his life. When William reached out to him for help, his father's primary mode of assistance was to berate and shame him.

His mother remarried when William was eleven. William describes his stepfather as being friendly and a good provider. However, William wondered if he wanted to pattern his life after his stepfather's. His stepfather worked at a job he hated for many years, yet as much as he complained about it to William, he would not take the risk of looking for another job. He also complained to William about his relationship with his mother, but he never addressed the reasons for his unhappiness with her.

Being a star athlete gave William entree into an exciting social life. After high school, sports continued to give him structure and meaning. Then, when he was twenty-nine years old, William had the motorcycle accident. He had difficulty throughout the rehabilitation process, not just because the physical therapy exercises were tedious and painful. His inability to move his leg with his accustomed strength and agility reinforced the reality that he would never be the powerful star athlete again. To accept that you are no longer able to operate at the same level of physical performance that you have been accustomed to makes for an extremely difficult transition.

William would alternate between self-pity and denial. Vicodin of course distorted both of these states. When he was feeling sorry for himself, he would cry in order to get others to pay attention to him. Self-pity is different from actual grieving. Self-pity is a recurrent means of distinguishing oneself by hopelessness and by hateful blame placed on others as well as oneself for personal tragedies. You feel that you have no choice but to submit to this hell, and you have no distinct plan on how you might move out of this quicksand-like state.

When you are stuck in the land of self-pity and denial, you refuse to take any responsibility for your problems. You are both clueless and fearful about what the possible solutions to your problems are. You are not feeling your real emotional pain. In William's case, he was feeling the pain of Vicodin withdrawal and physical pain from his accident.

William reports that during the early phases of therapy, he both lied about and minimized his prescription drug use. He informed me much later that his Vicodin use graduated to a more powerful drug, OxyContin. OxyContin gives you a sense of euphoria similar to that from high-grade heroin. William's heavy drug use distorted his thinking; it convinced him that he was managing his life beautifully. However, when he came down from the drugs, he was mean-spirited and nasty to be around. He lied to his wife, friends, parents, siblings, and physician about his drug usage. He would tell them he was in recovery when he was actually using heavily. He would become angry if those close to him confronted him on obvious discrepancies in his stories.

Withdrawal from drugs like Vicodin and OxyContin is far from easy. The symptoms that William experienced each time he attempted to stop using were constant tiredness, hot/cold sweats, heart palpitations, constant pain in joints and muscles, vomiting, nausea, uncontrollable coughing, diarrhea, insomnia, and depression. The recovery process from drug addiction is slow and fraught with relapses. Still, William has now accepted the need for the 12-step program of Narcotics Anonymous. He has a sponsor and attends meetings almost daily.

William's business is thriving, and his relationship with his wife has gone through a positive transformation. He realizes that his desire to be a "people pleaser" was part of his downfall, so he no longer looks outside himself for life-affirming answers. He is able to keep his personal life separate from his professional one and is selective when it comes to sharing intimate details of his life. He wants to understand and work through his fears in order to find the means to accept his physical limitations. He is optimistic that all his dreams can come true.

In my work with these clients, I was wondering if the incorporation of utilizing exercise along with self-questioning would be a more effective method than traditional talk therapy. I was curious if this method would work for others as it had worked for me. I also believed that I was developing a program that could be utilized as a self-help program rather than working with a therapist. I was excited about the possibilities.

Chapter Five

The Major Aspects of Exercise's Healing Power: Preparing for the Body-Mind-Soul Solution

The major aspects of exercise's healing power are:

- Increased self-esteem
- Increased mental and physical strength
- Improved mood
- Reduced stress
- Improved physical health.

That exercise improves physical health is commonly understood by most people today. The United States Surgeon General's 1996 Report on Exercise found that regular physical activity improves health by reducing the risk of dying prematurely, lessening the chance of developing colon cancer, and helping control weight, among other things. People with chronic disabilities can improve their strength and stamina both physically and mentally, by exercising regularly. At the same time that exercise reduces stress, it also improves mood; and the more that the healing power of exercise is realized, the greater grows your self-esteem.

Helpful as it is to realize the benefits of all five of these aspects, it is not necessary to do so before you begin the Body-Mind-Soul Solution. Focusing on any one of these aspects can prepare you for this program and provide access to your own healing power.

A fundamental component of the major Body-Mind-Soul Solution lies in the physiology of the bran. During exercise, physiological changes occur in the brain that enable you to deal with emotional pain at the same time you are working out. This chapter will examine those physiological changes and discuss their relation to the benefits gained through the healing power of exercise.

Endorphin, Serotonin, and Norepinephrine

The brain's neurotransmitters, chemicals that send out signals from the brain to all parts of the body, play an integral role in the realization of all the major aspects of exercise's healing power. The three neurotransmitters especially affected by exercise are endorphins, serotonin, and norepinephrine.

Endorphins can both relieve pain and effect feelings of euphoria (commonly known as the "runner's high") during prolonged exercise. Endorphins can also lower blood pressure and suppress appetite. Dr. Steven Keteyian, program director of preventive cardiology at the Henry Ford Heart & Vascular Institute in Detroit, has found that after only fifteen minutes of intense exercise, endorphin levels are increased. He says, "Whether or not the increase in beta-endorphin is solely responsible for the elevation of mood remains controversial. Regardless, we do know that exercise is an excellent approach to improve mood and treat depression."

According to Edward Laskowski, M.D., a physical medicine and rehabilitation specialist and co-director of the Sports Medicine Center at Mayo Clinic, "Endorphins are the body's natural pain relievers. Endorphins have the potential to provide the pain-relieving power of strong pain medications, such as morphine."

A recent press release from the Society for Neuroscience states, "New studies indicate that regular exercise may protect against Parkinson's disease or reverse some of the devastating consequences of traumatic brain injury. Other studies have found that, contrary to an earlier report, exercising alone appears to be as beneficial as exercising with others, and that the natural mood-enhancing chemical beta-endorphin may be a key player in the ability of exercise to protect the aging brain."

Serotonin is the neurotransmitter that adjusts mood, sleep, and appetite. Low levels of serotonin have been deemed to be the cause of clinical depression. Such new drugs as Prozac, Paxil, and Zoloft have been created to treat this illness by increasing serotonin levels. So does exercise. Indeed, Psychobiologist Henriette van Praag, Ph.D., declares that "Exercise has been shown to increase levels of serotonin in the brain. One could speculate that exercise is beneficial for depression by activation of the serotonergic system and/or production of new brain cells."

"It is easy to speculate that when you exercise, there is a change of serotonin system in the brain that could be affected and improve symptoms of depression," says psychiatrist Madhukar Trivedi, M.D., of University of Texas Southwestern Medical Center in Dallas.

A recent study by the British Journal of Sports Medicine supports this speculation. "Physical activity has the same effect as antidepressants," explains Dr. Fernando Dimeo, who led the research. "Aerobic exercise stimulates neurotransmitters in our brain to produce serotonin which makes us feel good. And exercise, unlike antidepressants, has no negative side effects."

The American Psychological Association states that norepinephrine is a neurotransmitter involved in our body's stress response. Exercise helps train the body to become familiar with experiencing stress. Furthermore, according to their studies, "Work in animals since the late 1980s has found that exercise increases brain concentrations of norepinephrine in brain regions involved in the body's stress response. Norepinephrine is particularly interesting to researchers because 50 percent of the brain's supply is produced in the locus coeruleus, a brain area that connects most of the brain regions involved in emotional and stress responses. The chemical is thought to play a major role in modulating the action of other, more prevalent neurotransmitters that play a direct role in the stress response."

The report also states that "Biologically, exercise seems to give the body a chance to practice dealing with stress. It forces the body's physiological systems, all of which are involved in the stress response, to communicate much more closely than usual:

The cardiovascular system communicates with the renal system, which communicates with the muscular system. And all of these are controlled by the central and sympathetic nervous systems, which also must communicate with each other. This workout of the body's communication system may be the true value of exercise; the more sedentary we get, the less efficient our bodies in responding to stress."

The effect that physical exercise has on brain chemistry is truly amazing. The changes in brain chemistry create the opportunity for the major aspects of exercise's healing power to unfold.

Increased Self-esteem

A significant aspect of exercise's healing power is the increase in self-esteem. Self-esteem is the degree to which one values oneself. If you have positive thoughts when you think about yourself and you are optimistic about your future, you have high self-esteem. Some indicators of low self-esteem are negative regard of your body image, negative thoughts about your character and personality, conviction that your aspirations will not come to fruition, avoidance of eye contact with others, and an unwillingness to take risks.

Many studies show that exercise increases self-esteem. While the subjects in such studies are various girls, boys, sufferers of chronic illnesses, substance abusers, the elderly, and adults without disabilities, results in all instances indicate that exercise increases self-esteem. A piece in the 1995 *Research Quarterly for Exercise and Sport* states that exercise has a positive impact on self-esteem. According to *Personal Trainer Magazine* published by IDEA (an organization of health and fitness professionals), in the year 2000 a review of the mental health benefits derived from physical exercise concluded that self-esteem improved with exercise and that people with low self-esteem showed the greatest improvements. Bill Phillips, author of the best-selling book *Body for Life: 12 Weeks to Mental and Physical Strength,* states that participants in his exercise and nutrition program have enlarged their self-esteem, confidence, self-respect, and empowerment.

The President's Council on Physical Fitness and Sports found that physical activity and sports boost self-esteem in girls. Girls also had improved attitudes toward body images and increased self-confidence because of exercise and sports.

J.P. Read et al. discovered that patients in treatment for alcohol abuse experienced an increase in self-esteem from exercising. In a study titled "Exercise Attitudes and Behaviors among Persons in Treatment for Alcohol Use Disorders," substance abusers reported that physical exercise raised low self-esteem. Fitness-Management.Com News asserts that exercise helps to improve health and fitness as well as boost self-esteem in older adults. In the August 2003 *Journal of Aging in Health*, researchers established that older women improved their self-esteem through exercise.

Broad research has also clearly established the positive effects of exercise on the self-esteem of people with chronic illnesses. One such study by Nakken et al. discovered that patients with epilepsy felt better in general and improved their seizure control with regular exercise. Another Nakken report concludes that exercise improves self-esteem and social integration regardless of its effects on seizure control. Segar et al. studied twenty-nine breast cancer patients and administered a battery of quality-of-life assessments after exercise training. The authors conclude that exercise improves self-worth, self-esteem, and mood status during and after chemotherapy for cancer patients. An article written by Russell D. White, M.D., with Carl Sherman in the April 1999 edition of *The Physician and Sportsmedicine* states that exercise increases the self-esteem of patients with diabetes.

Bob's Story

I'd like to share something of my own personal history to show how I discovered the value of exercise in improving my self-esteem. It was 1976, and my main form of exercise was lighting Marlboros and making mixed drinks with vodka (remember those sweet-tasting Harvey Wallbangers?). I was twenty-five years old and directing a program for runaway kids in Wichita, Kansas. I was obsessed with doing a good job. I worked, partied hard, ate McDonald's fish sandwiches for lunch, and slept only when I couldn't avoid it. I was also developing a gut way out of proportion with my skinny frame. I remember one stoned/drunken evening actually standing on a scale and being shocked that I weighed nearly 175 pounds. I was the guy known as "Bones, " the one who never broke 135. It was clear that I was extremely out of shape, both mentally and physically.

I had started smoking when I was fifteen and was now going through nearly three packs a day. I'd been athletic up to the time I entered college. I'd liked being active, and while I played sports in high school, I was never a "star" as I didn't really push myself to excel because I was so afraid of failing. By the time I hit my mid-twenties, I had not really exercised for a few years. I believed that sports were for kids and professional athletes. Real adults did not work up a sweat. Real adults were sedentary creatures who lay in front of the TV for their entertainment.

I had some idea that I was in bad shape, and I wanted to find out how strong my physical strength and stamina were at this point in my life. One day, I decided to go for a run around the block. I found some old sneakers, put them on, went outside, and was nearly blinded by the sunlight hitting my eyes. I started my version of jogging, which at that point was just a step beyond crawling—and I was gasping for air. I also felt faint, as if the oxygen of rural Kansas was unable to reach my brain. I could not even make it around the block before I was exhausted. I was also humiliated and shocked at how poorly I had performed. And I was still having a difficult time catching my breath. I did not share this experience with anyone, including my very supportive wife.

I have used many illegal drugs in my life, including pot, hash, LSD, Mescaline, assorted downers, and uppers. I also experimented with opium and heroin (snorted, not injected) for a short time. None of these drugs proved to be as difficult to quit as cigarettes. Cigarettes are both physically and psychologically addictive. To no avail, I had made literally hundreds of attempts to stop. I was finally able to end my dysfunctional relationship with tobacco only after I began exercising.

This occurred when I was unceremoniously fired from the runaway program because I was trying to prevent some members on the board of directors from stealing funds. It was a perfect time to begin a workout program. I was deeply worried about my future, and I now had time to focus on something other than my job. I played basketball every day at the Y with some guys who liked to exercise during their lunch breaks. After the basketball game I played a set of tennis with my wife. I never pushed myself too hard. I broke a sweat, but was never exhausted.

I was now exercising two hours a day, five days per week, and I was feeling stronger. Along the way, I quit smoking. My lungs were starting to clear; and for the first time since high school I could taste my food. My jump shot improved, and I was getting to the ball quicker during tennis matches. I was beginning to feel better about myself. I wasn't overjoyed with my very being, but my self-esteem was definitely on the upswing.

The ability to exercise on a regular basis increased my self-esteem on several fronts. As I had followed through on my commitment to get healthy, I could now follow through on figuring out what was going to be the next phase of my life. The toning of my muscles and my increased stamina led me to believe that hope existed in the universe. I began to have faith that I could grow on a personal and professional level.

I realized that while I was playing basketball and tennis, I was in a calm mental state that allowed my thoughts to clarify and my feelings to emerge. With the increased self-esteem that I gained from exercise, I was able to experience the emotional pain of being fired and face the fear of an uncertain future. I decided to apply to graduate school for social work. A few months later, I was accepted at the University of Kansas's School of Social Welfare.

Increased Mental and Physical Strength

Another benefit of exercise's healing power is the increase you can experience in mental and physical strength. You get excited when you find you can run farther and faster than last week. You feel immense joy at your ability to bench-press more weight. You are relieved that your blood pressure is dropping and happy that the pounds are falling off. You feel empowered because you are no longer exhausted at the end of your workout. You remember the great effort it took to get out of your easy chair, and now you are amazed that you bike two miles almost every day. Meanwhile, your mental strength is increasing as your brain's health improves; your thinking sharpens, and your memory is remaining acute rather than declining as you age.

Dr. Joseph A. Buckwalter states in *The Physician and Sportsmedicine* that regular exercise can slow or reverse the decreased mobility that can lead to chronic illness or disability in old age. Muscle loss, joint stiffness, ligament failure, and injury propensity can all be slowed or reversed through a regular exercise program. Indeed, exercise enables you to stay physically strong as you age.

A recent study by Mello et al. of bone marrow transplant patients indicates that exercise helps increase muscle mass, even in patients with chronic lower back pain. One can assume that increased muscle mass leads to increased physical strength.

Researchers from the University of Chester, UK recently completed a study on a group of women who participated in a resistance-training program called Bodymax. The purpose of the study was to assess the effects of a light, high-repetition resistance-training program on body fat percentage and muscular strength in women. The research indicates that these women increased their muscular strength.

Numerous studies show, too, that exercise enhances mental strength. A University of Illinois study compared two groups of healthy adults: one group did only stretching and toning exercises and the other group participated in aerobics. The aerobicisits improved performance on cognitive tests by 15 to 20 percent. The stretchers saw no gain. Arthur Kramer, who led the Illinois study, states that aerobic exercise such as jogging, swimming, or brisk walking three to four times per week will generate new brain cells. According to a 2002 study by J. Brisswalter et al., exercisers displayed improved decisionmaking abilities and improved cognitive performance.

Exercise does indeed keep your brain strong and prevent memory loss. *Fitness News* writer Shelly Drozd reviewed two recent studies that demonstrate the ameliorative effects of aerobic and strength-training exercises on the health of the brain and memory as you age. Unfit people tend to experience shrinkage of more brain tissue than do those who are physically fit.

"The biological changes prompted by exercise improve our capacity to master new, and remember old, information," says

Dr. John J. Ratey, Harvard University professor of clinical psychiatry and author of *A User's Guide to the Brain*. Ratey explains that physical movements call upon many of the same neurons that are used for reading, writing, and math; so it is perhaps not surprising that physically active people reported an increase in academic abilities, memory retrieval, and cognitive abilities.

The benefits of exercise in regard to mental strength are realized not only by adults; it also is beneficial for children. In 2006, the California Department of Education concluded, according to State Superintendent of Public Instruction Jack O'Connell, "Being physically fit is not only healthier, but studies have shown it can lead to higher academic achievement. It is up to us to provide ample opportunities to get them moving and motivated. Schools have the responsibility for providing standards-based physical education instruction, families can participate in regular physical activities, and communities play multiple roles in meeting the physical activity needs of children and adults," O' Connell concluded.

Bob's Story

I was twenty-seven when I entered graduate school. I was also unaware how truly confused about life I really was. I did not fit in the world of academia, and I began escaping its pressures in familiar ways. Cocaine was popular at that time; I did my share of snorting. I felt on edge much of the time. I felt I needed to get grounded.

I didn't exercise regularly when I first arrived on campus

because the demands of homework allowed me little spare time for recreation (except for recreational drugs). Occasionally I played basketball with my classmates, but it was not much of a workout. Meanwhile, most of the classes bored me to tears as I failed to find relevancy in most of them. I did not feel that the classroom was a good substitute for real-life experience. I was definitely an elitist in my own distorted kind of way. I nonetheless managed to do fine in school, even though I partied constantly. I became president of the social work student body—amazingly, since I did not know the first thing about running a meeting. Reviewing *Robert's Rules of Order* felt like reading an architectural manual.

Although I was in emotional turmoil much of the time, I landed the perfect job. I became an outreach counselor to teenagers at the local mall in Topeka, Kansas. One of my coworkers gave me an old pair of track shoes, and somehow they fit perfectly. I put them to use. I got up early one morning and, wearing some old sweats, walked over to the indoor track at the field house. I set my sights for running a half mile. I remember feeling that I'd not got much of a workout at that distance, so I ran another half-mile. After that, the sweat was running down my face. This seemed like a huge accomplishment.

I continued to run on a regular basis. I found the regimen gratifying and soothing, even though Kansas is not the best state for exercising outdoors since the temperature drops to several degrees below zero in the winter and hovers in the low 100's during the summer. Still, I managed to run a mile or so every other day.

Light though the training was, it made me feel stronger both physically and mentally. This sense of improved strength enabled me to ask questions about my life that I had not previously addressed effectively. I was able to focus upon issues like where I was going to live after graduation, what kind of career I wanted, what I wanted to be when I grew up, how much partying I should do, and how good I was as a husband and a friend.

Improved Mood

Exercise has been found to decrease the symptoms of anxiety and depression. While everyone experiences the effects of these emotional states, some people suffer them more intensely than others do. The number of Americans who evidence some form of anxiety is staggering. In 1998, the National Institute for Mental Health found that 19.1 million people suffer from some sort of anxiety disorder: 2.4 million have panic disorders, 3.3 million have obsessive-compulsive disorders, 5.2 million have post traumatic stress disorder, and 4 million suffer from generalized anxiety disorder.

Richard Cox, who headed up a research team at the University of Missouri Columbia, found that physical exercise significantly reduces anxiety. The team also discovered that the more intensely participants exercised, the sharper was their decline in anxiety over time. A recent study at the University of Central Oklahoma compared a sedentary group to a group that completed a sixty-minute aerobic activity. The active group reportedly had a greater sense of well-being and less anxiety than the sedentary group. According to the American Council on Exercise, "Exercise can help you feel less anxious. Exercise is being prescribed in clinical settings to help treat nervous tension. Following a session of exercise, clinicians have measured a decrease in electrical activity of tensed muscles. People have been less jittery and hyperactive after an exercise session." Researchers in Turkey studied 311 university students who had never taken part in any physical activity in their lives. They found that both males and females had decreased anxiety levels after exercising.

Depression is an illness that strikes many Americans. According to the National Institute of Mental Health, approximately 19 million adults suffer from depression. In addition, 2.5 percent of children and up to 8.3 percent of adolescents have been diagnosed with depression. The Institute also found that depression increases the possibility of having heart attacks in the future.

A number of studies reveal that exercise is an effective tool in reducing the symptoms of depression. An article in the April 2003 *Complementary Health Practice Review* shows that both aerobic and non-aerobic exercise are helpful for treating depressed adults. Another review of recent exercise and depression investigations titled "Exercise and the Treatment of Clinical Depression in Adults: Recent Findings and Future Directions" finds that although many of these studies have methodological limitations, there is a wide body of supportive material to show that exercise reduces depressive symptoms in healthy and clinical populations. University of Wisconsin psychiatrist John Greist and his colleagues have found that exercise reduced moderate depression more effectively than psychotherapy. A 2000 study of

3,403 adults in Finland found that those exercising at least two to three days per week were less depressed than those who did not regularly work out.

Is exercise as helpful for depression as medication is? Two recent Duke University studies beginning in 1999 have found that thirty minutes of brisk exercise three times a week is just as effective as drug therapy in treating those who suffer from major depression in the short term. In the long term, continued exercise reduces the possibility of the illness returning. Likewise, a 2001 *British Journal of Sports Medicine* pilot study found that exercise worked faster in reducing depressive symptoms than did medication.

Bob's Story

During the summer of 1979, after I graduated from social work school, the state of Kansas was undergoing a particularly ungodly heat wave. I had dreamed of living in San Francisco ever since my mother, sister, and I vacationed there in 1969, when I'd been charmed by the stunning landscape and the city's open acceptance of different lifestyles. So my wife and I packed up the car and drove to the city by the bay. Neither of us had jobs lined up, but we did have friends we could stay with and we had two thousand dollars to live off of.

I could not believe my good fortune to have ended up in San Francisco. The physical beauty of the place was a welcome sensory treat after staring at the emptiness of the Kansas plains for ten years. I was excited and ready to get on with my life. My wife and I spent countless hours availing ourselves of the wonders of the city: the Golden Gate Bridge with the fog rolling through it; the glories of Golden Gate Park; the richness of the cultures in the Mission, Chinatown, and North Beach, and the smell of the ocean's salt water. At the same time, I was job-hunting, and work was not plentiful in the late 1970s. I picked up the *San Francisco Chronicle* every morning and immediately applied for every social service job listed. The rejection letters piled up; I began to worry, and then I started feeling hopeless.

I finally was living in a place that felt like home. I'd never really felt this way when I was growing up in New Jersey or going to college and graduate school in Kansas. San Francisco had perfect weather, its politics were akin to mine, and there was so much to do. After our second month in the city, though, I began to fear that we would not be able to stay because I could not secure employment. I started applying for any kind of job; manager of a convenience store, temporary employment counselor, city directory salesperson. I didn't land any of them either.

I needed to find a way to deal with my topsy-turvy emotional world. I would get exhilarated that I was able to obtain a job interview only to be devastated by the rejection letter that seemed inevitably to follow. I was afraid to spend any money and really did not want to abuse credit cards. I was terrified that I would have to leave California and move to a state like Kansas that had more employment opportunities. The prospect was tantamount to taking a direct route into the depths of hell.

My wife found a teaching job soon after we arrived. That took off some pressure, but not a whole lot. My identity as a man revolved around what I did for a living. When people asked me what kind of work I did and I replied that I was unemployed, I could feel the dread flooding up in my heart. I remember times I'd stare blankly out the window, and see nothing, just a sense of total powerlessness because I was jobless.

I realized that I was both anxious and depressed. My constant feelings of fear and worry, along with a sense of impending doom, were symptomatic of my anxiety. My depression lay in my intensely hopeless thoughts and feelings. I had difficulty sleeping through the night, which I attributed to both anxiety and depression.

But I still had my former coworker's leather running shoes, and I decided to make use of them, although I was not consciously setting up exercise as a way to alleviate anxiety and depression. I wanted to combat boredom; I was tired of being home so much of the time without a job to occupy me. I put on the shoes, an old pair of shorts, and a sweatshirt. I remember that first run. It was cold and foggy. I ran around our apartment complex. I could smell the variety of ethnic foods being prepared for dinner; I heard the languages as various as the scents. I was so happy to be living here; I begged whoever was in charge, whether it was God, a Goddess, or the mayor of San Francisco, to make arrangements so I could stay.

We live near Lake Merced, and I began running there three times a week. This activity had a significant impact on my mood. Whatever worries or discouraging thoughts were troubling me before my exercise would have dissipated dramatically by the time my run was over.

During this period, I was regularly waking up around three

a.m. with visions of a U-Haul truck parked at the front of the apartment while workmen loaded our possessions into it for a move to Kansas, Nebraska, or Oklahoma—some place more remarkable for its frequency of tornados than cultural diversity or intellectual stimulation. At times, I was so convinced I was going to be banished from the Bay Area and I found myself crying into my pillow. My runs helped me to gain perspective. I reasoned that after all, I had only been living here a couple of months; eventually I would find a job. First I had to meet people who would give me a chance in this very competitive job market. While I was running, I also imagined the day when I was finally hired: I immediately would drive to Tower Records and buy a couple of albums. I was used to buying a few albums a month—sometimes a week—and I was definitely suffering from music-purchasing withdrawal though I don't think that this has yet been identified as a mental health issue.

One day, after an interview, I received a call from the Head Start Program in Southern Alameda County offering me a job. I accepted immediately. I celebrated by going out for a run and then driving to Tower, where I bought one of my favorite records of all time, Van Morrison's *Into the Music*.

Reduced Stress

Stress can be experienced physically as well as emotionally. It not only manifests itself as tension, worry, or apprehension, but also in stomach cramps, neck and shoulder aches, headaches, and other physical discomforts. When you feel pressured, stress is initially experienced in the brain, which releases adrenaline, cortisol, and other hormones. The release of these hormones serves as a precursor to uncomfortable or emotionally painful episodes. According to some research, half the patients who seek medical treatment for body aches are actually suffering from some type of psychological distress.

Shawn Talbott, Ph.D., writing for *American Fitness Magazine*, states, "In addition to exercise making you 'feel' better, exercise can change the way your body responds to cortisol. For example, an acute exercise bout will elevate your cortisol levels, adherence to a regular exercise program will 'teach' your body to produce less cortisol in response to a given workload." Many members of the fitness and mind-body community feel that the healthy effects of the brain's neurotransmitters—endorphins, serotonin, and norepinephrine—counteract the stress hormone cortisol during exercise. However, there is no concrete evidence to back this assertion up.

Emotional stress is a huge issue in this country. The American Institute of Stress estimates that one million people are absent from work each day due to stress. The National Institute for Occupational Safety and Health has determined that job-related stress is a major problem in America, where 40 percent of the work force finds their jobs extremely stressful. A 1996 *Prevention Magazine* survey found that nearly 75 percent of its respondents felt great stress on a weekly basis. A recent *American Heart Association Journal* report indicates that emotional stress causes heart attacks and may increase the risk of cardiac death.

The Copenhagen City Heart Study concludes that individuals who reported experiencing high stress levels are more likely to have strokes than those who did not.

Exercise reduces emotional and physical stress. A 2002 study completed by Dr. Rod K. Dishman, a professor of exercise science at the University of Georgia in Athens, found that physically fit women might be better able to fight off stress and therefore be protected against high blood pressure later in life. A 1999 *Annals of Behavior Medicine Report* found that exercise protects against the rigors of daily stress. Research participants who exercised reported having significantly fewer physical symptoms during periods of high stress. Exercise helps people get their minds off day-to-day issues that stress them out. It also revitalizes them.

High blood pressure is often caused by lack of exercise and too much daily stress. In the October 2001 issue of *Medicine and Science in Sports and Exercise*, researchers found that exercise, especially when combined with weight loss, reduces high blood pressure for people experiencing either high or low to negligible levels of stress.

Bob's Story

In early 1984, when I was working for the Head Start Preschool Program in San Francisco, I became involved in organizing my co-workers to join a union because the administration of our local version of one of the last Great Society programs was inept and unusually cruel to its workforce. The effort I was putting into my job was totally unappreciated by the administrators. As a result, I was frustrated, angry, and filled with stress almost every waking hour. In my view, the Head Start Program could have been an essential vehicle for organizing low-income folks into fighting against the creeping gentrification of San Francisco. But the people who ran the program certainly did not see it my way. They viewed their jobs as a way to increase political gain or as a means to get paid without doing any work.

My stress manifested itself as tightness in my neck muscles. At one point, my neck was as tight as the most severely tied knot. I could not move it without severe pain and needed muscle relaxants to loosen it up. I then suffered from one of the drug's side effects, agitation. I am sure that I was just a joy to be around.

The winter of 1984 was abnormally cold and wet in San Francisco, and another way that my stress manifested itself was in a series of upper respiratory infections. No sooner had one cold left my body than another arrived. I became alarmed that I could not shake this incessantly recurring cold, a response that only exacerbated the emotional stress I was already feeling.

Once the colds and tightness in my neck lessened, I increased my running mileage to five miles per day, five days per week. This routine did indeed help to alleviate my stress. It also helped me focus on my future. I realized that I could not work at Head Start much longer unless I was willing to accept the realities of community-based program bureaucracy and ignore the injustice all around me, and I knew that I was not willing. I'd have to leave.

I began studying for my second attempt at the state clinical social work written and oral exams. I'd flunked the first time because I hadn't taken them seriously. Once I passed them and obtained my license, private practice would become an employment option. I was learning that I did not deal well with authority, especially with bosses who were more concerned about covering their asses than performing.

While I was studying for these exams, I began training for my first marathon. I finished the San Francisco Marathon that July in three hours and thirty-seven minutes. The day before Thanksgiving, I received my new clinical social work license, ensuring that one day I would be working for myself. I have been a psychotherapist in private practice for almost twenty years. I still love it.

Putting Your Discoveries to Work

The flow of certain brain neurotransmitters released during exercise connects you with one or more of the major benefits of exercise's healing power. While you are working out, feelings of self-reliance lead to a sense of inner safety. This is an ideal state in which to use self-help psychotherapy techniques to heal your emotional distress.

The self-assurance gained from experiencing one of more of the major benefits gives you the impetus to explore the causes of internal wounds. Increased self-esteem provides the courage for you to begin looking at painful thoughts and memories. Increased physical and mental strength enables you to face the painfulness in your journey by self-discovery and to realize that you will not just get through it; you will be a more complete person for it. Improved mood affords you the faith that painful memories can be transformed into peace. With your experience of reduced stress comes the desire for increased happiness by overcoming emotional pain. Your quest to improve your physical health opens up the pathways to resolving the hurt inside.

You are ready now to embrace the Body-Mind-Soul Solution.

Chapter Six
The Body-Mind-Soul Solution

Y ou are now ready to begin the Body-Mind-Soul Solution. Before you begin your first workout, review the following list of possible questions to ask yourself while exercising. The questions come from the Emotional Pain Questionnaire in chapter 3 and from the investigations of emotional pain in chapter 4. Feel free to create your own questions as well.

Questions to Ask Yourself about Physical Symptoms that have been ruled out as physical problems only by your physician

- Why am I feeling headaches?
- Why am I experiencing muscle aches?
- Why am I experiencing rapid heartbeat?

111

- Why do I get stomachaches?

- Why am I grinding my teeth at night?

- Why do I have sleep problems?

- Why do I have a lack of energy?

Questions to Ask Yourself about your Current Emotional State

- Why am I easily agitated?

- Why do I have difficulty enjoying activities that once held great interest?

- Why do I have difficulty getting along with others?

- Why have I been crying more than usual lately?

- Why am I feeling emotionally numb?

- Why do I feel disconnected from others?

- Why do I have difficulty thinking clearly?

- Why do I have difficulty concentrating?

- Why am I worrying so much of the time?

- Why am I afraid to stand up for myself?

- Why don't I give myself credit when I do well?

- Why do my feelings get hurt so easily, and why am I unable to soothe myself?

- Why do I have difficulty trusting others?

- Why do I have difficulty forgiving others?

- Why do I have difficulty forgiving myself?

- Why do I have low self-esteem?

- Why do I have difficulty making and maintaining friendships?

- Why do I have difficulty making and maintaining intimate relationships?

Questions to Ask Yourself about your Childhood History

- How was I affected by being abused by my parent(s) or others close to me?

- How was I affected by being neglected by my parent(s) or others close to me?

- How was I affected by being emotionally abused by my parent(s) or others?

- How was I affected by being sexually abused as a child?

- How did my parents' lack of play time with me affect me?

- How did my parents' unrealistically high expectations or low expectations affect me?

- How did my grade, middle, and high school life affect me?

- How did my parents' discipline methods affect me?

- How do I deal with failure?

- How did my parents' praise affect me?

- What was the most positive event of my childhood?

- What was the most upsetting/traumatic event of my childhood?

Questions to Ask Yourself about Stuck Grief

- What does stuck grief feel like?

- Why is it so hard to resolve?

- Does listening to music while exercising help break through this emotionally constipated feeling?

- What memories does music stimulate?

- Am I angry with someone? What for?

- Do I feel that I was abandoned at some time in my life?

- How does it feel to have been abandoned?

- If I could have a conversation with the person who abandoned me and/or hurt me, what would I say?

- What would I want this person to say to me?

- Am I able to cry about this loss? How does it feel to cry?

- Am I angry about what happened?

- What needs to happen so I can feel better about this loss?

Questions to Ask Yourself about
the Death of a Loved One

- What was the person who died like?

- What do I miss most about him/her?

- How does this loss affect me?

- Do I feel that no one understands my pain?

- Do I have difficulty expressing my feelings about this loss?

- Do I worry about my own mortality?

- What have I learned from this loss?

- Am I having difficulty getting close to others because of this loss?

Questions to Ask Yourself about The Teenager Within

- Does my anger often prevent me from achieving my goals?

- Do I feel a sense of anguish when I am disappointed?

- What is this anguish about?

- What were the most significant events of my adolescence?

- Do I feel that my life is filled with drama?

- What is that drama about?

- Do I sense that I have a teenager within?

- What is he/she like?

- What kind of facial expression or body language does he/she have?

- How does my teenager within express his/her hurt?

- What does my teenager within need in order to ease his/her pain?

- Who was emotionally available to me when I was a teenager?

- What was I like as a teenager?

Questions to Ask Yourself about Anger that Hurts Those You Love

- Have I ever been verbally abusive toward anyone?

- Have I ever been physically abusive toward anyone?

- Have I ever wounded anyone with my words?

- How did I feel immediately after abusing/wounding someone?

- How do I feel about it now?

- Do I feel guilty or ashamed?

- How did my words affect my loved one?

- Why do I think I have been abusive?

- How does this abuse begin? What is the cycle?

- What comes first: anger or hurt?

- Do I feel entitled to be abusive toward my loved one?

- Do I have problems managing my anger?

- Do I beat up on myself in the same manner I beat up on my loved one?

- What can I do to alter my abusive behavior?

Questions to Ask Yourself about The Ancestors Anguish

- How do I feel about what my ancestors experienced?

- How does their experience affect me?

- Do I feel that I have any behaviors or feelings that stem from my ancestors' plight?

- How do I feel about being (your ethnicity)?

- Can I look inside myself and get in touch with any of my ancestors?

- What are they like?

- Do I have any questions for them?

- Can I describe their anguish?

- What can they tell me about genocide?

Questions to Ask Yourself about Investigating Emotional Pain

- Why do I have obsessive rituals?

- Am I in denial about how major life crises have affected me?

- Why am I in a state of denial?

- Do I minimize the effect major life crises have had on me?

- Why do I minimize?

- How has my family's substance abuse affected me?

- How has my substance abuse affected me?

- How has the fact that my parents never talked about their feelings affected me?

- How has longing for the approval of others affected me?

- Why do I have panic attacks?

- When do I have panic attacks?

- What triggers my panic attacks?

- What am I afraid of?

- Did I ever place my mother or father on a pedestal where they could do no wrong?

- What happened to cause them to fall off that pedestal?

- Why am I codependent?

- How does being codependent affect me?

- Why do I push away people I care about?

- What do I turn to when life becomes overwhelming?

- Why do I push away or push down my anger?

- What happens when I push away or push down my anger?

- Why am I estranged from {insert family member}?

- Why am I afraid to be alone?

- Why do I have problems with commitments?

- Why do I have nightmares?

- Why do I tend to evade emotional pain by working constantly?

- How did I feel when I couldn't relieve my parents' misery?

- How did I feel when my brother or sister hurt me?

- Why do certain memories make me feel sad?

- Why do I feel that I cannot count on anyone else to help me?

- What were the unwritten rules in my family, and how did they affect me?

- Did my anger ever get me in trouble?

- Has my intense responsibility for someone else ever caused me problems?

- Have I become more determined to help someone after my efforts were dismissed? If so, why do I feel this way?

- Is there something I feel very guilty about? What is the source of that guilt and why have I been carrying it around for so long?

- Do I have a physical illness or injury that I am having difficulty coming to terms with?

- How has a parent's mental illness affected me?

- How has violence in my family affected me?

- Does my emotional pain affect my parenting? How?

- What provides me with a sense of control? Is this healthy?

- Do I allow people to take advantage of me? Why?

- Do I meet the societal expectations of what a man/ woman is supposed to be? Is this a positive or negative aspect of my life?

- Do I have difficulty reaching out to others for help?

- Have I ever stayed in a relationship long after I should?

- Have I noticed negative similarities between my partner and my parents? Why is this so?

- Do I become very emotional when I hear a certain song? Why is that so?

- Do I have issues regarding personal boundaries? What are they?

- Did I have to deal with bullies when I was a child? How did this affect me?

- Do I feel free? If not, what will it take for that to happen?

What if I Am Having Problems Identifying what Troubles Me?

This is OK. In fact, it is very common to have difficulty identifying what is bothering you. One of the primary reasons for this difficulty is that people who live in dysfunctional families consider the behavior they see on a daily basis to be normal. For example, a twelve-year-old girl who picks her drunken mother up off the floor each night and helps her to bed might think that situations like this are common in most families, especially if the child is forbidden to talk with anyone about her parent's behavior.

It is also possible that you have learned to distance yourself from emotional pain. Let's go back to our twelve-year-old girl. As a survival mechanism, she pushes away the fear, panic, and disgust that accompany the burden of her alcoholic mother. She utilizes a defense known as compartmentalization, whereby she stores all of her distressing memories in the unconscious recesses in her brain.

Or perhaps you come from a family in which the expression of emotion was simply not allowed. Your parents may have expected you never to utter an angry or sad word, and they may have punished you if you did otherwise. You may still be carrying this parental demand inside of you.

What can you do if you know something is bothering you, but don't know what it is? Go to your computer or grab a piece of paper and pen. Write down all of the important events in your life, both positive and negative. Make a list at first, then go back and elaborate on each item on it. There is an excellent chance that this process will help you find what troubles you.

I find writing to be particularly helpful to me when I'm trying to discover the source of my emotional pain. For example, in my attempt to deal with residual teenage pain, I wrote the following in my journal:

> It was the beginning of the summer of 1969 and the ceremony took place in the stuffy school gymnasium. I did not feel the effects of the humidity because I was high. My friends and I ate a few marijuana brownies and our brains became mush-like. I had trouble walking to the stage and receiving my diploma. My grandparents and mother were appalled at my physical condition. Later, I was deeply ashamed of my behavior and felt like the future was going to hurt me.

I then developed a series of questions based on this entry that I would ask myself while exercising: "What was my last year of high school like?" "Why did I choose to get so high that day?" "Why did I go out of my way to embarrass my family?" "What was my self-esteem like in high school?" "Why did I feel that I had no future?"

During one of my workouts I explored the question, "What was my self-esteem like in high school?" The result appears in this journal entry:

> I am listening to Patty Griffin's "Tony," which is a sad song about a gay teenager who ends up killing himself because he felt so hated. I feel the sense of teenage alienation that this song focuses on. It is a rock-and-roll song filled with loud guitar and brittle lyrics. I feel the angst inside as I head out the door. I start to run slowly and my joints seem to creak with each step. I think about a therapy session I had with a high school senior yesterday. I connected with his sense of alienation from his peers. The scenes from my painful memories emerge as I pick up speed. I remember feeling put down by the more popular kids in high school. I wasn't smart or athletic enough for their sensibilities. I was never going to be as successful as they would be. I have spent the last 30 years or so trying to prove them wrong. I suddenly realize that my attempts to prove them wrong aren't solely motivated by trying to gain their approval. I am also trying to undo the past and recreate history. I want to erase all childhood memories of being humiliated by peers, teachers, bosses, and coaches. I want all that pain to evaporate into the stratosphere, but those memories refuse to leave.
>
> My legs and arms pump in unison as the music of loss and love pours into my soul. These hurtful memories have been my enemy to slay in battle. The pain of rejection has driven me to push past the scornful faces that did me wrong.

The bitterness protects my vulnerability as it weighs me down
and keeps all that is fluid stuck. I feel an ache deep in my
stomach as I watch my legs go harder and faster. All I wanted
as a child and a teenager was to be accepted and loved by my
community. I felt ostracized by the entire town. I fantasize that
a tickertape parade in my honor takes place on a sunny day in
my hometown. Everyone is standing along the street cheering
my name. I realize this will never happen as I sprint the last
quarter mile of my run and then cry.

In this session, as the journal indicates, I got in touch with one of the main reasons why my self-esteem suffered during adolescence. I realized that I had never felt like I fitted in and this realization helped me understand why I had acted out so much in high school. As I ran, I experienced again the sadness that the isolation had brought when I was in my teens. I had never really felt it that deeply before.

This exercise/self-questioning session led to further exploration into my teenage years, and I continued to grieve over a time in my life that was hurtful and disappointing. Through this process I was able to eventually let the ugliness in these memories go and move toward loving myself.

BEGINNING YOUR WORKOUTS

This program is designed for anyone who regularly engages in running, jogging, walking, biking, aerobics, Rollerblading, or similar individual sports. Physically, your workout will differ in no way from what you usually do. Your warm-up and stretching routine will not vary.

During your first workout in this program, start with the question that resonates with you the most. For example, if "Why am I experiencing stuck grief?" speaks to your current concerns more than "Do I have problems managing my anger?," focus on your grief.

It is better not to ponder whatever question you choose before you begin your workout. It is important also to assess your mood and the way your body feels as you begin, because you want to prepare yourself for looking inward. Write down this assessment in your journal (see appendix), along with your emotional pain question.

Before you begin your first workout, be sure to have a "safe place" inside yourself, somewhere you can go to if your feelings become too charged or frightening. Visualize a peaceful scene like a beach at sunset or some other place you associate with tranquility. If your feelings do indeed become too frightening, immediately go to your "safe space" until the intense emotions subside.

Journaling after the workout is a crucial part of the program. It is important to journal as soon as a workout ends so that you can capture the sense of well-being you have obtained doing your exercise. Writing down the thoughts, feelings, and memories you have experienced while working out will assist you in remembering the lessons you've learned about emotional pain. It will help instill these new beliefs, ideas, and insights into the core of your being. It will enable you to expand on these lessons and thereby deepen your understanding.

It is possible that this program will bring up painful feelings that may prove to be overwhelming, and you may need counseling to deal with them. It is essential to have the name of a therapist available just in case.

Performance

Start asking your emotional pain question as soon as the workout begins. The technique you will be using here is known as looking inward. Its aim is to make you more keenly aware of your thoughts, feelings, mood changes, and the external environment. Notice how you feel at the moment you begin to exercise. Are you concentrating on the question? Is your heart beating faster? How is your breathing? Is it smooth or belabored? What is happening around you? Has your pace begun to increase? What other thoughts and feelings are you conscious of?

Sandy G., a 50-year-old Jewish woman who lost her mother eight years ago and her father last year, provides an excellent example of looking inward. She chose stuck grief as her emotional pain topic, reviewed the possible topic questions, and decided to ask herself during her first workout how she felt about her mother's death. She wrote in her journal:

> *Why is it important that my mother be proud of me? Why does it make me feel like a better person, woman, mother, if what I do is something she approves of? How upset will my children be when I pass away? How do I deal with the fact that I will never*

see my mother or father again? Why do we love our parents no
matter how displeased we are with them?

Alice W. is a 29-year-old woman who lost her father to cancer
nearly two years ago. She was very close to him. She looked inward and wrote:

> *The music of the Indigo Girls and Melissa Etheridge along*
> *with the sun makes my heart swell. I feel so happy. When I feel*
> *like this, I sometimes feel guilty or surprised. I wonder how*
> *I can feel so happy when I haven't seen my dad in so long,*
> *when I miss him so much. I remember the first time I felt really*
> *happy after he died. It was at a local lake with friends and*
> *we were having so much fun eating, swimming, and relaxing.*
> *I realized that although I had truly thought I would never be*
> *or feel happy again, I did. And I cried out of the relief that life*
> *can go on.*

As you can see from the examples above, the initial emotional pain question triggered additional inquiries. It is important to this process that you allow the questions to flow and not
worry about answering them. The more liberally the questions
increase, the more readily you will tear down the walls that have
prevented you from facing your emotional pain in the past. This
is a very freeing experience.

New insights and revelations come quickly and often in this
program. These new perceptions will lead you to a deeper

understanding of your pain and perhaps eventually lead to the resolution of it. The revelations in themselves are exciting, thought provoking and reassuring. They may occur at any time in the beginning, middle, or end of the session. Always be receptive to them.

When you have an emotional pain insight, tell yourself to continue thinking about it. Let the thoughts and feelings linked to the insight come forward. Notice how you are feeling while all this activity is progressing. Remind yourself to write the insight in your journal when you have completed your workout.

Rhonda G., a twenty-six-year-old African-American woman, chose The Ancestors Anguish as her emotional pain topic. She entered this revelation in her journal:

My ancestors live on and they give me strength. During college I had a picture of Jesse Owens that I carried to all places I traveled where I was the "only one." As a long distance runner, often times I found myself being the "only one." Certainly, in most of my college classes, graduate classes, and law school classes this phenomenon kept repeating itself.

I think my resiliency stems from learning about my ancestors. Not only did I learn about them, but I believe in race memory and so I believe I know them. Knowing my ancestors, recognizing their integrity has transferred to me, is powerful.

Running calms my mind and serves as a break from the hostility I encounter in so many spaces and places. I sometimes ask them, "How did you do it and how did you survive"?

Fifty-two-year-old Laurie G. wrote this revelation:

My father died four years ago and I have a difficult time
grieving his death. I feel guilty, but that was the theme of my
adolescence to feel guilt, take the blame and full responsibility
for the tumultuousness of our relationship. My father
undoubtedly struggled with the fact that I would never be like
him and he feared my uniqueness. The guilt I carried was like a
poison that erodes self-confidence and joyfulness. I was existing
between my mother and father largely because they were unable
to communicate with each other. I was the sole source of their
happiness; stuck right in the middle. They were complacent
as long as I did not cause any disturbances or take chances. I
learned to always stay within bounds, to not ask for too much
because I was taught that I did not deserve anything.

This dynamic affected me deeply. I have the ability to see
two sides to every argument, but have difficulty taking a stance,
a valued opinion. The message I got from my parents was that
they did not care about my feelings. I was afraid of my father's
anger and it was better to be silent than confront him.

The Body-Mind-Soul Solution enables you to release your
emotional pain; you will feel it happening. Be aware of the sweat
streaming from your pores. Experience the sweat as emotional
pain leaving your body, as if you can feel, see, and smell the angst
exiting and letting go.

During one of my workouts, I had intense memories of the
ten-year period I was a cigarette smoker, from age fifteen to

twenty-five. Smoking was a difficult habit to break. After I finished my run, I wrote in my journal:

> *Sweat is pouring out of all my pores. I feel all the tar and*
> *nicotine that I forced into my lungs from age 15 to 25 pour*
> *out of my body and onto the street. The cigarette juice is dark*
> *and gooey. I hear my body thank the runner in me for expelling*
> *this murderous substance. I don't want to die. I want to win.*

Another technique to effect emotional release is to deal with anger as it arises in the course of your workout. Many of us do not know how to deal with anger. Either we attempt to repress it, to force it into silence, or else we have inappropriate outbursts. In this program, you can run to the anger as well as through it, as Laurie for example did.

She wrote:

> *As I ran and listened to music as a teenager, I could run farther*
> *away from my father's anger. Perhaps this emotional pain*
> *suppressed my very being and smothered the spontaneity that*
> *life offers. Today the music allows me to run faster, perhaps*
> *attempting to run through the barrier of anger instead of away*
> *from it. Maybe I will eventually run through the shame.*

Another example of dealing with anger as it arises in the course of your workout is found in the following journal entry of Lucia J., a forty-five-year-old Mexican-American woman from Los Angeles. She was originally introduced in chapter 4; having a very difficult relationship with her sister Silvia. Lucia is married and has no biological children. She did raise one of her former lover's children, however. This child is now twenty years old with a child of her own. Lucia had parents and four siblings who lived nearby; they are all now gone. Lucia recorded the anger she experienced as she recalled it working out on the treadmill:

I have actually been thinking about what are the causes for my anger long before I jumped on the treadmill today. I am angry for a lot of reasons. Funny, one of them is being angry at not being angry. I always discount what is or what has happened to me. Just shoved it right down because other people's problems or feelings were supposed to be more important! Where the hell did that come from? Why do I do this? I am angry because I have been taken advantage of by so many people in many ways.

Some of this was my fault because I chose the wrong people or situations. But, I understand that I was lost and looking for things I was not getting. I'm angry because I never had a family connection. I always felt a distance except with my sister Deena. I am angry that my parents have not had the chance to see what I have become. I am angry that I lost my father, the one person I felt who really loved me even though at times he couldn't understand me. I am angry that I grew up surrounded by drug use that was never addressed. I am angry that I am losing my brother whom I was just beginning to feel comfortable with after all this time. I am angry that no one ever assisted me with progress or growth, that I was never

encouraged. I am angry that now at age 45, I should be 30—
just beginning. I am angry that my circumstances have led me
to start my life late and I feel that I am running out of time. I
am angry because for the first time in my life I feel happy deep
into my soul and now I feel deep sadness like a blanket over
that happiness. I want to feel that way again. Lord, I hope I
feel that way again.

Sadness, like anger, can be effectively dealt with during a workout session. Experiencing the sadness, recalling and examining it is another efficient emotional release technique. Often we deal ineffectively with sadness; we tend to push it away by denying it or else holding on to it. Denied or harbored, sadness can lead to feelings of depression and being stuck. This program enables you to face the reasons for the sadness.

The sadness may be experienced during the actual workout or while journaling afterward. If you recall a sad experience while you are exercising, you may begin to cry and/or feel yourself sink into despondency. Your re-experiencing of this sadness may then trigger further related memories that together afford you new insights that will help ease your despair. It is important to remember what occurs during this process so you can record it in your journal later. As you recall and write down the powerful emotions you have experienced during the workout, you may have additional insights regarding the sadness; insights that will increase your confidence when facing emotional pain.

Sandy G. located the origin of her sadness at holiday times in her mother's death. She wrote:

> I start to think about the long holiday weekend coming up
> and wish I could spend it with my mother. I miss not having
> a mother, who cared more for you and your kids than anyone.
> It was a different type of caring than you receive from your
> husband or friends. I start thinking if I were able to see her and
> speak to her for one hour, what would I say? Imagine seeing,
> feeling and smelling her after eight years. Just the thought of it
> has me welling up.

Cheryl O., a thirty-year-old El Salvadorian woman devastated by a failed relationship, wrote:

> I am trying to get over my last relationship and the painful
> breakup. There is no sense of closure and the fact that we don't
> speak to each other, makes it harder to move on. I feel that I have
> wasted 3½ years of my life and I will never get them back. It's
> so hard because once again, I've been let down. The one person I
> cared about, that I loved turned his back on me and left when I
> needed him to be there. This will be a long road for me.

The imagination can also offer a means for facing emotional pain. While you are exercising, use your imagination to script an imaginary meeting between yourself and the person with whom you have unfinished business. Picture the person in your mind.

What would you like to say to her/him? What would you have liked her/him to say to you? You can't change what actually happened, of course, but by imagining what could have happened, you will summon up lots of feelings about what happened and perhaps arrive at new insights into a long troubling situation.

Cheryl O. wrote:

One of these days I need to write a letter to myself. I need to tell myself that I am a great person, that I have so many wonderful qualities, I have so much to offer and one relationship, one man, is not going to change this. I've written so many conversations in my head about what I would do if I ran into him. I would want him to apologize. I have to make peace with myself one of these days and it is going to be up to me because this apology is not going to take place.

A voice recorder can also be helpful with the Body-Mind-Soul Solution. I decided to purchase a small digital voice recorder because I was finding it increasingly difficult to remember all the important thoughts and feelings I was experiencing during my workouts. The longer you work out in this program, the more intense becomes the experience. In my case, the thoughts, feelings, belief questioning, and insights were coming so fast and furious during my runs that it was impossible to recall them completely for my journal. Using the voice recorder relieved the pressure of my trying to remember everything that was happening to me emotionally and intellectually during the workout. Now, when my run is over, I go to the computer, open up my journal file, listen to the voice recorder, and write down what I hear. I find I frequently put the device on pause so that I can write down insights that occur to me as I'm transcribing the tape.

Listening to music while working out is another option you may want to include in the program. Your choice of music can, to a significant degree, determine your exercise pace, influence your mood, and affect your energy level. Purposely chosen, the music can also invoke memories from your distant or recent past. The recollections it prompts may in turn help you to recognize and face various aspects of your emotional pain. The music indeed may "speed up" the process of recollection and recognition by inducing memories that may not otherwise occur without it.

Reading your journal entries a few hours or days after entering them will give you a sense of your progress. It may be helpful when reviewing your journal to highlight the most meaningful thoughts and feelings so that you can strategically formulate questions for your next workout.

You have now begun the Body-Mind-Soul Solution. You are formulating questions and utilizing them during your workout. You have started to face your emotional pain. This program can take you farther, beyond new insights to discoveries.

Chapter Seven
Discoveries

The Body-Mind-Soul Solution can bring you to one or several discoveries even in your very first session. Among the kinds of discoveries you can expect to glean from this program are:

- New insights about your emotional pain. Once you begin to learn the origins of your emotional pain, you will find new ways to process it. Discovering insights, then, is a major step toward resolving whatever is troubling you. Your insights will support your hope that you will in time find all the pieces of your trauma puzzle. Your insights will motivate you to continue investigating your emotional pain.

- The ability to face emotional pain without distraction. By focusing on your emotional pain during your workout you can expedite the healing process. Perhaps the main obstacle to healing emotional pain is the fear that arises when you initially concentrate. The fear prompts you automatically to stop processing your pain and allows you to become distracted by other thoughts. When you are exercising, however, the changes in your brain chemistry enable you to overcome the fear of facing your personal trauma. The anxiety surrounding your emotional pain suddenly vanishes or else is experienced as background noise. Each time you experience the retreat of fear, you will be able to delve deeper into the origins and memories of your emotional pain.

- The ability to experience anger and sadness fully. Not only will you come to understand the origins of your emotional pain, you will be able to recognize and deal with its effects. Another hindrance to working through emotional pain is the inability to give the appropriate expression to two of its debilitating effects: anger and sadness. Often we either bury our anger and sadness inside ourselves or express these emotions in an abusive fashion. Our open encounters with anger and sadness tend to be brief. The combination of questions that address emotional pain with exercise permits you to more fully healthily experience anger and sadness in a fluid, uninterrupted way. You will be able to feel the sadness come up through your body as the tears run down your face. At the same time you are experiencing the rage, you will be understanding the reasons for it. You will feel yourself letting go of the anger or sadness as you increase the pace of your exercise and the flow of perspiration from your body.

- The capacity to find your wisdom. As you let go of your emotional pain, you will begin to find your higher self and to access the place inside yourself that holds for you constructive truths. You will enter your personal palace of wisdom. Some call this place the psyche; others call it the higher voice, or God. It is the place you can go to when you feel lost, confused, and in need of answers. Most of us have been taught that the answers we seek during our personal crises exist only externally to us; that someone or something holds the key that will release us from suffering. Many of you beginning the Body-Mind-Soul Solution may not have ever yet accessed your place of wisdom because of childhood abuse or some other trauma that has barred your belief in yourself. When you hear your internal voice of wisdom speak, you can trust that it is speaking your truth. Trust and accept. Acceptance is the final stage of the process of working through emotional pain. Acceptance doesn't mean that you will now forget everything that caused you pain. No, you will always remember the bad things that happened to you. However, when you wholly accept that they have, you will no longer struggle internally with them. You will no longer question who or what is responsible for hurting you. You will instead allow yourself to surrender to your truth. For example, when I finally, after twenty-five years, accepted that my father was dead and was never going to return, however much I suffered or hoped or agonized, the huge black cloud that had hovered over my head for decades at last began to dissipate.

- The ability to use the power of your imagination. Scripting an imaginary scenario about a bad memory can be, in itself, an effective mode of healing emotional pain. When to this imaginative play you add exercise, an emotional pain question, and music, you have the elements to occasion significant change. In my journal entry titled "Happy Birthday to Us" (which is included in the next chapter), I conducted an intense imaginary conversation with my father. Now I want to be clear—I was very well aware that my loved one was no longer with us. This is not about being delusional. While you may feel silly with the "make believe" aspect of this process, it is worth overcoming your inhibitions, because the healing power of imagination can be strong and immediate. In my case, I created the space inside me for my father's spirit to enter, and he "spoke" to me.

To illustrate how these various discoveries might occur during a workout session, I'm going to share some of the journal entries made by a woman you were introduced to in chapter 4 and met again in chapter 6; Lucia J., a forty-five-year-old Mexican-American woman trying to make sense of the multiple losses she has experienced throughout her life.

Workout #1

Type of exercise: Treadmill

Length of Exercise: 30 minutes

Kind of Emotional Pain: Healing Stuck Grief

I looked up the definition for tragedy today. The third definition was "a disastrous event; especially one involving distressing loss or injury to life." The fourth was "a tragic aspect or element." The first was "a drama or literary work in which the main character is brought to ruin or suffers extreme sorrow." Why do people assume that tragedy and drama are part of the same? Those of us who experience tragedy do not see ourselves as the starring role in a drama or literary work. In fact, we have no control over the drama our lives have turned out to be. I always said if I wrote a novel, no one would believe it was the truth. It would all seem so unreal, and many times to me it feels the same way also.

How can one deserve so much pain in their life and to have so much pain and loss that they do not know how to accept others' love or understanding? Isn't it sad when all you know is rejection, survival, and dependence on yourself? When you just start to learn how to become someone who lets others in, you again become lost in that constant sea of grief that constantly overcomes you. It is not a feeling of depression. No, for you know that all too well. Climb into your cocoon; surround yourself in darkness, for it makes you feel safe. Keep your distance and no one or nothing will hurt you. Hide your fears, for only the strong survive.

Grief, well, that is something totally different. According to Webster's, the definition of grief is "a deep and poignant distress caused by or as if by bereavement." Well, that was interesting, so I looked up *bereavement*: "the state of being bereaved; especially in the loss of a loved one by death." So I looked up *bereaved*: "suffering the death of a loved one." Suffering; that does not touch the enormity of the feeling that you feel. There is NO definition of the feelings that you experience. The loss, the emptiness, the guilt, the profound sadness for what you lost and, at the same time, what you did not have. The loneliness accompanied with the fact that you will never share an experience with the person who meant so much to you, no matter how volatile your relationship. It is hard to put day-to-day life into perspective when your world as you know it has disappeared from the face of the earth.

I was the last child in a family of six children. I am now 45 years of age and am the only survivor of my family. I have experienced a profound loss, not once, not twice, but seven times over, eight if you count my grandmother, who was a large influence in my life. I did not only lose them, but I seemed to lose them in groups. It started when I was 21. My mother died on April Fools Day; how appropriate for her. The doctors only gave her three months to live when she was diagnosed. She joined an experimental trial for Methotrexate before it was approved, lasted one year, and passed away on April Fools Day. I always thought she was snubbing her nose at her doctors. Every time I see Methotrexate used now, I know my mother made a difference, even as she lay dying, to change someone's life.

A year and seven days later, my beloved Grandma, who probably saved my life by taking care of me every summer, died. I was lost. I was attached to my aunt who was also there every summer. We would drive to the beach in her Impala with the plastic-covered seats. Knowing that after spending the day, we would come back up to the car and burn our seats on the plastic. She came to the river every summer, her and my uncle. They would bring my cousin, who was her grandson, and we would live a carefree life; at least in those summer months. He, too, came from a place where there were lots of problems. Auntie taught us how to swim, slowly giving us confidence in ourselves. We knew we had made it when we could swim across the river to "the log" or to the tree swing, where all the big kids swam. Sometimes we would even swim upstream to sit in the rapids, or row the boat in front of the beach. God, how those years saved me. I used to feel like I was just shipped away, gone the day after school let out, and I did not return until the day (literally) before school began. Now, I know that those summers just may have been the only grace in my life. They saved me, probably my cousin too, for that was the only time I understood routine, sanity, and love. Interestingly enough, I also lost my aunt. She did not die, but because I was so young and did not understand what was happening in my life, I thought if I stayed close to her, I would lose her, too; so it was easier to distance myself, than to lose someone else I cared about.

I went to school, partied too much, and really did not apply myself, as I could have. No one cared, so why should I? I do not blame my parents, for they did the best with what they had. I was literally a mistake—one of my siblings made sure that I knew that. Funny, the one who was most dependent on me and the one I felt most obligated to care for. My oldest brother was 15 when I was born, the youngest 9½, there were 5 of them, twin girls after the oldest, then two boys, then—oops—me.

In 1990, my brother Ted died. He bled to death from esophageal varices at the hospital. As long as I can remember, Ted had a drug problem. He was always in trouble for something. I can remember always going to jail waiting in line to see him or to another prison. Most kids played on the weekends, not me; I went to see my brother. I loved Ted. I understood too that he loved me. He always called me his little girl. I can remember seeing him detox for the first time when I was about 9. Funny, I knew what was happening, but somehow no one wanted to address it. In 1992, my brother Simon passed away during a liver transplant. You know, I vividly remember calling my brother Pat at the firehouse and telling him he needed to go and tell my dad. I could not tell him again, that someone had died. Even though my dad was a policeman, the night my mother died he came and woke me up and told me I better go and check my mother. He was a policeman for 30 years, still slept in the same bed with her throughout her illness, yet I had to tell him that yes she was gone. I am sure he also knew that it was me who took her oxygen tubes away at her request. I asked her if she knew what she was doing, what it would mean, she said yes, and so I followed her wishes. Ted came home and told me she had her oxygen off. I told him that was what she wanted and she died shortly after.

In 1994 my father, who was the light of my life, died. It was on a Saturday night. There was a party for my brother Pat's 50th birthday. My father had told us days before, when he was still aware, that he wanted us to go, carry on as usual. My father was moved out of the ICU that afternoon, he was disoriented and calling out to people who had passed long before him as if he was greeting them on the street. I knew in my heart that he was on his journey and truly had already left us. I leaned over to say good-bye to my "Papi." He had been so disoriented, yet when I said good-bye and that I would see him later, he pursed out his lips to give me one last kiss good-bye. That memory lives on in my heart. Every so often, when I awake in the night and cannot get back to sleep, my lips will automatically purse out, and a feeling of peace comes over me and I am able to return to sleep, knowing somehow that he is by my side.

In 1996, my sister Dolores, the burst of sunbeam, the person who taught me to enjoy life, had her gall bladder removed. Strange things happened and slowly she was taken away from us. She was removed from life support. I can remember standing at a window outside the Neuro ICU with Pat and Deena. My comment, "and then there were three…" freaked them both out. But in the end, it was the truth.

I never dealt with the losses that I experienced, just drank to numb the pain. My mantra was "live each day as if it were your last" because in some ways, that summed my life up. I was very destructive, any way I could be. I did not allow people to get to know me, did not choose good men, drank, and partied like there was no tomorrow, because for me, the chance was there would not be. I was all about the moment. Forget the future; how could one have a future when nothing was expected of them and no one really cared, especially myself, about what happened to me. I let myself be enveloped in the shroud of darkness that could be comforting as a blanket at times and so, so lonely at others.

I met my husband during these traumatic times. We were on, we were off, but the most important thing was somehow we were. I can still tell you what he was wearing when I first met him. He, too, was running away from demons. He fortunately realized he had to deal with his demons and, in saving himself, threw me a lifesaver that saved me as well.

JUST when you think you're doing well, WHAM I lost my sister, and then four months later my brother died. My sister gave up on life. My brother struggled until his very last breath to live life to its fullest. It is these two events that I will try to focus on, for it is the first time I have experienced the grief process as it is happening. I am not only grieving for Pat and Deena, but for Mom, Gramma Tina, Ted, Simon, Delores, and my daddy, who I miss each and every day.

Slowly, with the help of an understanding grief counselor, with my husband who has experienced loss in his life, and with my belief that I can survive, I have begun my road to recovery.

Lucia discovered the origins of her emotional pain and found new ways to process it. Having gained the insight that facing her emotional pain could be healing, she mustered the courage to tell the story of her multiple losses. She asked herself, "How can one deserve so much pain in their life? So much pain and loss that they do not know how to accept others' love or understanding?" She did not shy away from answers of the further questions that presented themselves. She grappled with her conflicting emotions. She learned to discern feelings of grief from feelings of depression. Whereas depression took her to a place inside that was dark and numb, she experienced grief as sadness, emptiness, guilt, and knowledge that she would never see her loved ones again. She realized, too, that she felt staying with her grandmother as a child had saved her life because it was the only time during her childhood that she enjoyed a family structure and love. She learned that distancing herself from others like her aunt, who was part of those good summers, was her attempt to protect herself from the pain of losing them.

These discoveries led Lucia to understand that she had turned to drugs and alcohol in order to numb her pain. She became self-destructive because she felt as though she was living on borrowed time. Now she realized that she was running away from her demons rather than facing them. When she recently lost her last brother and sister, she had the insight that she had never before experienced a "normal" grief process and this time she was going to work through her losses, but just not those of her brother and sister. She was now mourning for all of the losses in her life.

In addition, Lucia learned how to experience anger and sadness fully, for she had resolved now to deal with the intensity and meaning of her grief as it was occurring rather than as a distant, hazy memory. She has examined survivor guilt, being the last family member alive. She has struggled with the unsettling fact that she had been allowed to live while her loved ones have perished. She has been able to get in touch with the profound sadness she felt over her father's death more than twenty years ago. While she was exercising, Lucia was able to confront the essence of her pain and choose not to numb it, as she had done in the past. And her guilt began to lift as Lucia began to understand that so many losses had made it difficult for her to maintain intimate relationships, although she has remained committed to doing so with her husband.

Lucia has found her higher self. She has found the will both to survive and to recover from her eight losses and the belief that she can. Lucia has learned that she can now face the reality that she will never see her lost loved ones again. She realizes that although her relationships with family members were often and in some instances continually volatile, she still loved them deeply. The truth was, Lucia discovered, that she would only let people get just so close before pushing them away. As a result, she felt increasingly isolated and alone. Lucia is now able to look at the loss of each family member separately and to view the losses collectively as well. While the gravity of her losses will continue to weigh on her, she knows that her burden will lessen if she continues to consciously grieve while working out. She had discovered the truth that death is part of life and that facing it is not as painful as pushing it away.

Workout# 2

Type of Exercise: Walked ¾ of a mile on the treadmill
Length of Exercise: 20 minutes
Kind of Emotional Pain: Healing Stuck Grief

The tears, the feelings, and all the emotions that have been locked up for so long hurt. What would I say to my mother? "Why didn't you love me?" I guess. I really want to believe that she loved me in her own way. I think deep down, she truly loved me; however, I could never stop thinking that because I was a "change of life baby," as I was reminded by others at times, that I was the cause of her depression. I changed her life, and somehow it was not for the better. She escaped by drinking and not letting herself get emotionally attached to me. No one really cared what I did, as long as I was home when I was supposed to be. No matter what I was doing, it did not matter.

How sad is it to not want to love your child? I remember hugs once in a while and how good that made me feel, but often after those signs of affection the distance came. Interestingly, I just now see the parallel. I too would let people get only so close and then push them away. Obviously, I learned well! Proof that children do learn what they live. Further proof is that I thought that turning to drugs or alcohol would numb my senses and my feelings, only to find that after the numbness I ached and was more raw than ever before.

It was strange to hear other people call her Ma or Mom, because many looked at her that way. She was available to them but not always to me, and I could never figure out why. Perhaps she thought that I was strong, perhaps she was afraid. These things I will never know.

I can say to her that I forgive her for not being available. That I feel sorry that she could not identify her illness of depression and alcoholism and feel that she could do something about either one of them. I would tell her that I love her and I miss her dearly. I wish that we could have had the chance to build on our relationship. I would like to think that as I got older that she would be proud of my accomplishments. I wish that we had spent more time together and gotten to know one another. I am sorry that I really did not know her. I know her characteristics. I know her a little bit but I did not know her.

I have tried to be a good mother to Rita. Funny, sometimes I hear my mother in myself. Depending on the situation, that could be a good or a bad thing, but either way, it always brings me into check.

The discussion I had with myself about my mother was very powerful. And in the end, things seemed less heavy, not like I was carrying something around. Even now, although I have tears running down my face, it is easier. There is no guilt that I was not good enough any more. I think I truly realize the depth of her depression, and her inability to love me had nothing to do with me but with her illness.

Wow, that is a heavy thought. Maybe I should just let things be and accept this as the answer, if there is really an answer.

Lucia now understands that her mother's inability to parent her had nothing to do with her. It was instead the product of her mother's depression and alcoholism. The Body-Mind-Soul Solution helped Lucia to face emotional pain without distraction and to focus on and expedite the healing process. She was able to tell the story of all her losses without being distracted by confusion, shame, or guilt. Indeed, she says at one point that she feels no guilt about her mother's life and death. The Body-Mind-Soul Solution's combination of exercise, focus on a particular facet of emotional pain, and journaling allowed her to concentrate with intensity and achieve a depth of realization that she hadn't known previously.

Lucia learned, too, the therapeutic value that lies in creating an imaginary scene about a bad memory. She imagined a conversation with her deceased mother in which she finally had the chance to ask, "Why didn't you love me?" In the interplay between imagination and memory, Lucia discovered she could forgive her mother for not being there for her and not being able to face her depression and alcoholism. Lucia could tell her mother that she loves and misses her.

Workout# 3

Type of Exercise: Treadmill

Length of Exercise: 30 minutes

Kind of Emotional Pain: Healing Stuck Grief

Mack and I just returned from a nice trip up the coast. We drove up the coast and watched the sunset sitting on a bluff overlooking the ocean. The colors were spectacular, the scene was beautiful. Who would have ever known I would be so lucky to experience such a sight or a feeling?

It was truly a long leisurely ride, restful, yet somehow I was not completely at peace. This will be the first Thanksgiving without Deena and Pat. While I did not spend many Thanksgivings with Pat, it seems empty to not have the usual disagreements with Deena about the holidays. This is a different type of stress I am feeling, and I am afraid that it is taking its toll on me physically. I was so happy to have some time with Mack. It seemed to bring us back together again, not that we were drifting apart, but the last 5 months have been difficult for me, to say the least, but have been, I feel, just as trying if not more, for Mack.

Lucia is now deeply mourning the recent losses of her brother and sister, but she is experiencing this pain intensely in the present rather than of as a distant memory. Furthermore, at the same time that she is examining how these deaths affect her, she is focusing on improving her relationship with her husband. To live in the present is the goal Lucia strives for, now that she has had a taste of its benefits.

Lucia's story is inspirational. It demonstrates how effectively the Body-Mind-Soul Solution can work in only a few sessions. In the program Lucia's motivation to heal found its means, and the more she dedicated her energies to the program, the more her resolve to get better increased. Her discoveries have been astonishing.

Chapter Eight
The Journaling Experience

Writing in your journals immediately after your workout will create further progress in your emotional
pain journey. Expanding upon painful and positive
memories you've recalled while exercising will make you feel
that you are growing mentally. Memories that were previously
hazy will now become clearer as you write them down, and you
will be able to heal the emotional pain associated with them.
Journaling also allows you to track your progress from one entry to the next and to reflect on the ups and downs of the healing process. Writing in your journal gives you the opportunity
both to record and amplify your music/exercise/emotional pain
question experience. Your entries will chart the course of your
journey toward total well-being.

The gifts to be gained from journal writing are evident in the
samples that follow. In some instances the participants worked an
emotional pain category; in others they were working through an

emotional pain question they themselves devised before exercising. Some of them listened to music while working out, others did not. You should do whatever you find to be comfortable and helpful to you.

If you are wondering how to begin your journals, notice the different approaches the various case study participants took as they entered the workout experience in their journals. Some immediately began writing about their emotional pain. Others focused mostly on their physical exercise. Still others integrated their thoughts about emotional pain and physical exercise both, along with observations regarding the music they were listening to. There are many different starting points. Choose any you find useful. What's most important is that it allow you to write freely.

Sandy G., who we met originally in chapter 4, is a fifty-year-old Jewish woman who lost her father and mother in the last decade.

Sandy G.
Workout #2

Type of Exercise: Spinning
Length of Exercise: 1 hour
Music: Funk, pop
Kind of Emotional Pain: Healing from the Death of a
Loved One

I am getting on my bike, adjusting it to fit my short frame. I start talking to the therapist next to me who is telling me about some of her clients. I proceed to tell her how I hate Mondays, as it is the start of the routine. I am pedaling as I speak to her to get my legs going and my cardio up. The instructor comes over to us to check our bikes, and he starts to tell us we will be going up three hills. I feel tired already, thinking I will not have the energy for this today.

I start to think about the conversation I had with my sister today about how she would like me to get more involved in the finances of my mother's estate. She tells me about the last moments of my mother's stay in the hospice and how my mom gave her the "death stare." I knew that was one of the reasons I did not visit my mom at the end because I did not want to remember her like that. I start to feel a cramp in my foot, as I am sure I am not pedaling correctly. I should slow down or even stop the bike, but it is starting to get better. We take a water break for 30 seconds and then start the next hill. I like this next song, but I have no idea who is singing it. This beat gets me going and I start to have more energy. I start thinking about how my sister is making me feel guilty about not being there at the end, for my mom, but I am sure it is my own guilt that I am feeling. My mom might have known I was there and I might have provided a great comfort to her. But maybe I was too selfish to visit her. I was just thinking about how seeing her would affect me, and not how she might have realized I was there and provided comfort for her.

I cannot concentrate on anything now but trying to reach the top of this hill. I have the bicycle on a 9, which is the hardest you can pedal, and I am so hot and my breathing is labored. It is time to go to the next level, and it is getting easier and easier. The last hill is over and it is time to cool down. I am now just concentrating on how fast the time went and how I need to relax and just take a shower.

Sandy G.
Workout #3

Type of Exercise: Kickboxing

Length of Exercise: 1 hour

Music: Funk, pop

Kind of Emotional Pain: Healing from the Death of a
Loved One

My arm is still sore from this weekend playing tennis, but I know once I start punching and kicking, I will forget the pain. I forgot my armband, which may present a problem. We are warming up with small punches and kicks and I am feeling good. I start to think about the long holiday weekend coming up and wish I could spend it with my mother. I miss not having a mother who cared more for you and your kids than anyone. It was a different type of caring than you receive from your husband and friends. I start thinking if I were able to see her and speak to her for one hour, what would I say? Imagine seeing, feeling, and smelling her after eight years. Just the thought of it has me welling up. I remember when she first passed away and how I would cry in the shower every night. A day did not go by where I did not cry, alone of course. I did not want to upset the kids, and I actually wanted to mourn alone without anyone asking me anything; without anyone looking at me wanting to hear about how I felt.

My arm is now starting to hurt, so I am taking the punching down a level. Funny, but when I start thinking about deep, depressing thoughts, my energy level is so high that I feel I am thinking clearer with more forethought. My thoughts just come streaming out without my worrying about not thinking about certain things because I do not want to depress myself. I miss my mom's voice and how she would be so excited whenever I called her. She was such a positive person and I am not. I also do not think about her every day as I used to. How upset will my children be when I pass away? How long will they think about me every day until I am an afterthought, and thought about, maybe, once a week?

I have to stop for water after this routine because I am so thirsty. I cannot imagine someone who has not gone through the death of a loved one to understand a loss of such magnitude. How do you deal with the fact that you will never, ever see this person again? How do you deal with the fact that you want to tell this person certain things in the course of a day; you want to share a joke, some gossip, that only this person will appreciate? I understand that it is a part of life to lose your parents and people you love, but I wish there was some manual to help you not be completely miserable when it occurs. How long will these feelings last? I think it will rear its ugly head forever. Time to cool down. I am so ready to go home and read a good book.

Sandy G.
Workout #4

Type of exercise: Kickboxing

Length of exercise: 1 hour

Music: Funk, pop

Kind of Emotional Pain: Healing from the Death of a
Loved One

I feel so rushed, getting out of work late, having three days off from work. I do not want to be here, but I am warming up and feeling the music. This instructor has so much energy; you have no choice but to get into it. I start thinking about how nice the weather is in New York and remember how my father would love this time of year. I again start to think how his wife killed him, how he was so unhappy, how he could never say or do anything to please her. I thought I would get over my feelings of antagonism toward my stepmother as I matured, but it only intensified. I was able to see what an unhappy woman she was and how she wanted my father to be something he was not. He was never going to make a lot of money so she would not have to work any more.

My kicking and punching is intensified as I think about my stepmother. He could never make her happy, no matter how hard he tried. No matter how hard we tried to convince him to leave her, he would not. Was it because he truly loved her and liked the abuse? Was he afraid of being alone? If only he left her, my sister and I feel that he would have finally had a good life. He would have moved to Florida and lived with my sister. He loved the weather and loved being around my sister. They had a special relationship, which in some ways I envied. I think because I am quiet just like him and my sister is outgoing, he enjoyed being with her more. I wonder how much this really bothers me.

I need a water break and my arm is seriously bothering me. I cannot stop tennis or kickboxing unless I am completely debilitated, which may be sooner than I think. We are finally cooling down, which is where I need to be right now. It is amazing how fast my workout is when I am not just thinking about my aches and pains; wondering when it will all be over and how close this person got to kicking me. I am feeling so strong and always so happy with myself that I was disciplined enough to complete another workout. I have to go home and take some Motrin, but I am still thinking about my father who, no matter how much he disappointed me, I still loved. Why do we love our parents no matter how displeased we are with them?

Regarding her workout #2, Sandy writes about the mode of exercising she is doing, the discussions with others in the gym, and the way she is feeling physically before she takes on the issue of her emotional pain. This task allows her to build up to the difficult issues she plans to face. When she does face her emotional pain, the endorphins may have kicked in, so that she feels safer addressing her parents' death. Sandy records the memories and feelings she experienced during spinning exercise, then focuses on her guilt about not having seen her mother before she died. Although this issue is not resolved here, it is important to note that Sandy admits to having avoided these memories since her mother's death. The Body-Mind-Soul Solution has given her the means to address the loss and the guilt. As she writes, she is now able to face the fact that she was too overwhelmed to visit her mother while she was deteriorating. She couldn't bear the prospect of watching her mother dying slowly right before her eyes. She was afraid. Hopefully Sandy will learn that this sort of fear and avoidance is not unusual and she will find a way to forgive herself.

Facing her mother's death, as she recounts it in her journal after workout #2, enables Sandy to have an imaginary conversation with her mother during workout #3. Sandy remembers being very sad after her mother died, but she kept these feelings to herself. Now being able to immerse herself in the memories of her deep connection with her mother, Sandy is able at last to grieve and to face the fact that she will never see her mother again. This is perhaps the most difficult issue to deal with when grieving the death of a loved one. The stark truth that you will never see that person again is immediately and intensely painful and scary, though eventually the awful pain yields to sadness, and ultimately to acceptance.

Sandy's feelings about the loss of her mother opened up the opportunity for her to grieve her father's loss in the next entry.

While she wonders if her father didn't leave her miserable step-mother because he either enjoyed her abuse or was afraid of being alone, at the very end of the entry she asks the question that many of us are compelled to ask: Why do we love our parents despite their shortcomings and our displeasure? Perhaps one day Sandy G. will find an answer.

Sandy feels that the Body-Mind-Soul Solution is very helpful to her. She has found it much easier to face her emotional pain while exercising than she did being sedentary. "Exercising is such a positive thing that allows me to focus on my painful emotions and at the same time gives me the opportunity to distance myself from them when they become too much to bear. I can be more positive and understanding of my parents while exercising. The thoughts and feelings come up around the reality that I will never see my mother or father again. This is extremely difficult to deal with. It was most difficult in the beginning when my mother passed away and at times it is still difficult to comprehend how I can go on. This pain is much easier to take in while exercising."

Frank M. is a fifty-five-year-old man who we met in chapter 2, whose father was a belligerent alcoholic. Frank's goal in the Body-Mind-Solution Program was to come to terms with his father in order to let go of the anger he felt toward him. He also wanted to examine the issues he had with commitment and intimacy.

Frank M.
Workout #1

Type of Exercise: Treadmill

Length of Exercise: 1 hour

Emotional Pain Question: What would I say to my
dad in a letter?

Dear Dad,

For so long now I have wanted to tell you how damaging you were to my development as a human being. As a young boy I can remember hunkering down in my bedroom for fear that you would come home from work in an alcoholic rage and start going off on me. It used to make me sick to my stomach when I would hear the ice from the icemaker tinkle into your glass. Many times, you would not even come in to say hello to me, which was at the same time ok by me and hurtful that you didn't care enough to see how I was doing.

I can remember eating dinner alone while Mom waited for you to come home because you were "working" late. Actually, we knew you were out getting drunk. I have often wondered how Mom could spend all those years waiting for you, knowing full well you were out getting drunk. When she would call you on it, you would become enraged and verbally abuse her.

I spent most of my formative years in survival mode, in constant fear of you. I grew up a shy, introverted, sensitive boy who had a really hard time interacting with other people. Being in a group was painful. It was so difficult for me to feel that I had anything worthwhile to say because I had such low self-esteem. Nothing good that I ever did was acknowledged positively. When I screwed up, though, the negative feedback was hurtful and relentless.

I remember feelings of hate as I grew older. I couldn't wait to move out of the house when I entered college. Once I was gone, I never wanted to come back. I felt like I never really got to know you and couldn't remember one meaningful conversation with you, or words of encouragement or advice.

I also want to tell you that my feelings about you changed when my wife died. You came over to the house the next day and hugged me and told me how sorry you were. You were so supportive during the funeral and afterward. It was a side of you I had never seen. After that, you spoke to me differently. It changed even more after your heart attack. I remember being in the hospital when they were wheeling you into surgery. I told you everything was going to be all right. You squeezed my hand tight and I saw real fear in your eyes. It was the only time I ever saw you vulnerable, and I felt a combination of fear and compassion.

Dad, I want you to know that I have forgiven you for the past. I realize now that your behavior was based on your upbringing, and I know you did not have an easy childhood. I have not been a perfect parent myself. I have been cold and unapproachable to my children. I have worked hard the past two years to become more approachable and open to them. Our relationships have improved immeasurably as a result. It is never too late.

Love, Frank

Frank M.
   Workout #2

Type of Exercise: Treadmill
Length of Exercise: 1 hour
Emotional Pain Question: What issues do I have
                        with intimacy and commitment?

I recently broke up with my girlfriend. We had a relationship of 3+ years. We broke up once about two years ago. The issue at that time was about conflicting expectations; she wanted to get married, I wanted a girlfriend to hang out with.

A couple of months later we reconciled. We agreed to work toward a common goal of progressing the relationship to the point we could both feel comfortable. We discussed a pre-nuptial agreement, living together, waiting two more years until her daughter graduated high school, even the possibility of marriage. Through it all, there was this continuous underlying discomfort that we simply did not want the same thing. We talked openly and frequently about the issues, but it always came back to one issue . . . she needed marriage to feel "honored." I felt myself withdrawing whenever the subject was broached.

Finally, we talked honestly about where we thought we were in the relationship. We concluded that we were really no further along than when we first broke up. I told her that I couldn't continue along in the relationship knowing that there was this ongoing pressure to deliver something I didn't feel good about. We broke up again.

Two weeks later, she called me and we met for dinner. She told me that she had started therapy and found a really good therapist. She said after one session she discovered that she was really in denial about some issues she had not dealt with growing up and felt that she was blaming me solely for having a lack of commitment and intimacy in our relationship. She said she felt she had been unfair by laying sole responsibility on me and that she was accepting her share of causing the relationship to be dysfunctional. She all but asked if we could get back together and try to work it out. It made me wonder if I really do have intimacy and commitment problems, or if the issues I raised were valid and she simply was not the right woman for me. It made me think about how important it is for me to trust my feelings and not be so quick to blame or question myself about decisions that I make.

The work that I have done regarding self-esteem issues has been important to my well-being. Before, I would have totally withdrawn or made a decision based on fear; the prospect of being alone, believing she was right and I was to blame, not feeling worthy. This time, I trusted my feelings and did not surrender to the old tendencies caused by low self-esteem. So now I am focusing on being clear on what it is that I want in my relationships. I realize no one is perfect, but there are certain things that are relationship killers. I would like to be in touch as to what those things are and to be aware at the beginning of the relationship so they don't become huge problems later.

I also would like to be clearer on whether or not something is truly a relationship killer or just an excuse to prevent me from commitment and intimacy. I know there is risk in any relationship and that so much of the other person's emotional state has nothing to do with me. I want to have the sensitivity and good sense to be open to the idea that I may have set unreasonable standards and have a willingness to explore all possibilities. I just don't want it to get to where I am doubting myself and making really bad decisions as a result.

Frank felt that his letter to his dad would provide the structure he needed to address his emotional pain. This is a very effective use of journaling. Writing letters to someone who has abused you is a long-established therapeutic technique that encourages you to express your true feelings without hesitation, fear, or inhibition since there is no expectation your letter will actually be sent.

Some people in fact do send their letters. In the letter format, Frank was able to call up memories that at one time he would have considered trivial, but that now brim with significance for him. Thus he realizes that in his memory of the ice tinkling from the icemaker into his father's glass lay deep emotional pain, for that tinkle was the prelude to the verbal abuse that would follow.

What was important for Frank was to clarify his thoughts, get in touch with painful memories, and let go of his angst surrounding his father, so he saw no need to actually send the letter. During his first workout he faced very painful memories without minimizing or rationalizing his dad's brutal behavior. He came to understand, too, that his difficulty in connecting to others was the direct result of his father's verbal abuse. Yet he also was willing to forgive his dad, he realized, because he now understood that his father's own awful upbringing had caused his violent behavior.

Forgiveness is an important element in letting go of the emotional pain. Understanding that our parents' own traumatic childhoods may have caused them to be abusive can lead to forgiveness; however, forgiveness is an emotional and spiritual process that takes time and effort. In his first journal entry, it's clear that Frank was ready to forgive his father. The progress Frank made in dealing with his father during the first workout enabled him to focus on his life in the present. During the second workout Frank gained the insight into his difficulty in separating his personal issues from those of others. In the past, when Frank's primary relationships were floundering, he would immediately blame himself for any problems without even considering that his partner might also be responsible. As he was working through the responsibility issue, he also realized more clearly what he wanted from a relationship.

For Frank, the Body-Mind-Soul Solution clarified issues that had been confusing him much of his life. He discovered the source of his low self-esteem. He found that he could value more fully himself and his opinions now that he acknowledged being mistreated as a child, a painful fact that he had spent years avoiding. He learned how to stand up for himself and to be assertive without being abusive.

James K., introduced in chapter 2, suffered from the abandonment of his father. When James was very young his father divorced his mother and made no concerted effort to be part of James's life after he left. In his journal, James explores how his father's abandonment has affected him.

James K.
Workout #1

Type of Exercise: Running

Length of Exercise: 1 hour

Music: Rock and Roll

Emotional Pain Question: Why am I so angry?

I'm feeling so rejected because I truly believe that my father didn't love me. In fact, I don't believe he ever loved me or he wouldn't have acted as he did. As I run, I feel a rush of emotion, tears well up in my eyes in the darkness. I run faster. Why didn't he ever fight for me? For me. I'm angry and dejected that he doesn't have the backbone to fight, the courage to venture into the unknown now or in the past. In fact, it makes me think that he doesn't know how to fight for anything. He walked away from Mom and he walked away from me—twice. He abandoned me once again. As I reflect, I think I only wanted to see signs that he loved me, a phone call, congratulations, a birthday card, but I never have and this is a source of emotional pain.

Not feeling loved by your father is a terrible thing. I know I have done nothing to deserve the treatment that I have received, but that doesn't ease the loneliness and isolation I feel. He is dead to me, but he is very much alive both physically and as a source of anger in my soul. I must eradicate him as a source of infection and pain. I need to abandon him so that I can remove the demons from within. But how? I want so much to be free of this anger. Can I find solace in the unconditional love I receive from my children and wife?

James K.
Exercise #2

Type of Exercise: Running
Length of Exercise: 1 hour
Music: Rock and Roll
Emotional Pain Question: Why am I so angry?

The anger my five-year-old son Johnny feels probably runs parallel to what I am experiencing to some extent. When I disappear to work, he gets so angry that I'm not there to love him. I, of all people, should have recognized this long ago. He needs his dad and his dad needs him. I guess the Beatles had it right when they sang "All You Need is Love." Perhaps the relationship that I forge with him will serve as a peacemaker for the demons that battle within my soul. Can I find peace by building the father-son relationship with Johnny that I never had with my dad? I don't know. I am, however, no longer fearful that I don't know how to establish this type of connection. I can and am doing it.

I feel personally responsible for the anger that Johnny feels at times. I know that I have shown more love for him than my father has ever shown me during my entire life. I tell Johnny I love him and I show him my love and affection. But then there are failures during times when I'm traveling or pouring myself into a work deadline. I am not there for him and I let him down. Why do I do this when I know how much it hurts? I feel like a failure as a parent during these times.

I have a small revelation as I continue to search for a means of understanding my father's actions. I don't believe that he is capable of love. Nothing he has ever done fosters the selflessness that love demands. I find that comforting. I have always searched for answers as to why he acted the way he did. I constantly run through different scenarios that never provided answers as to why he acted the way he did, but served to fuel the anger inside of me because this is no acceptable explanation. If he is incapable of love, then he is not rejecting me. Can it be that simple? I hope that I am not fooling myself because I don't want to. But as soon as I thought about his inability to love, it made sense to me. At least right now, I find this soothing.

James immediately delves into his emotional pain issue in both of his journal entries. He recounts that he runs early in the morning, while it is still dark outside; as soon as he faces the pain of his father's rejection, he begins to cry and run faster. Increasing your speed during your aerobic workout enables you to dig deeper into the origins of your pain. It also further builds confidence in your ability to work through personal trauma. While James had been angry much of his life, he was not aware of why he was filled with rage. In the first workout, as he writes in his journal, he faces the awful truth that his father didn't love him. It's a truth he avoided most of his life, although he has always been terribly confused about his feelings for his father: He couldn't understand why his dad never reached out to him.

In the past, James protected himself from this painful truth by either denying or avoiding the father issue. Instead he would take out his anger on his wife and oldest child. Now, while he is exercising and focusing on his anger, he is able to deeply grieve his loss. Throughout much of his life James had wondered if he'd done something to push his father away; if he'd had some character flaw that made his dad despise him. Now James truly believes that he was not in any way guilty or responsible for his father's behavior.

During the second journal workout, he experiences a soulful connection between himself and his oldest son, Johnny. He realizes that at times he, as a father, has been distant from Johnny, but he recognizes, too, that he is capable of being a loving father. James, on the other hand, is incapable of love, and in his acceptance of this sad truth James finds solace.

Shortly before beginning his journal, James arranged a meeting with his father, to whom he had never before really talked about his deep anger. Although his father had long been absent from his life, James did see him at family gatherings, and his stepmother always sent his kids Christmas presents. When they met, James asked his father to stop sending the presents and informed him that he wanted to formally terminate their relationship. His father did not argue or protest; neither did he shake James's hand when he left. Father and son experienced no meeting of the minds. In the first journal entry, James asks, "Why didn't he ever fight for me? For me." He is wondering still why his father made no attempt in James's childhood and more recent past to establish a loving, close relationship with him. In contrast to his father who walked out on him, James affirms his desire to be a present, loving father to his son. He has found the pathway to healing his emotional pain.

Laurie G., who was introduced in chapter 6, is a fifty-two-year-old woman who dealt with complicated issues regarding her parents.

Laurie G.
Workout #1

Type of Exercise: Running
Length of Exercise: 45 minutes
Music: Lauryn Hill, Eurythmics
Kind of Emotional Pain: The Teenager Within

I am aware that a layer of emotional tension resides deep within my body. I struggle with this tension, which I view as a lingering shadow that obstructs and suppresses. This tension resides within the core, entering my being. Often my feelings range between disappointment, anger, grief, and doubt. Not deserving, failure, fear. But strenuous exercise has always been calming and nurturing to my spirit, alleviating layers of stress grounding my emotional misdirected tensions. I process my anxieties and worries as I run. Silenced throughout my adolescence, the fear of speaking, getting attention, has suppressed my ability to own visibility. Silence is a pervasive presence held by unconscious memories. I am aware of anger. Poor parenting, unsupportive, discouraged. Differences and eccentricities frightened my family so they stifled my individuality, creating a doubt that left me fearful and doubting my self. Unable to embrace difference propagates fear and hate—like the war, oppression is fueled by ignorance and hatred. Trust in self. My body aches, my chest is full.

Laurie G.
Workout #3

Type of Exercise: Running
Length of Exercise: 45 minutes
Music: Diana Krall, Only Trust your Heart,
        Joan Osborne-Relish
Kind of Emotional Pain: The Ancestors Anguish

Reemergence and transformation. Reemerging a stifled spirit. The dark. Feminine suppressed. Women have been silenced throughout time, perpetuated into a dark abyss, struggling to be heard and visible. When I run, I repeat the lines from an Audre Lourde poem *So it is better to speak, remembering, we were never meant to survive… we were never meant to survive… we were never meant to survive.* The collective unconscious speaks to the feminine, the shadow of doubt represents the thousands of years of collective feminine suppression, gender and sexuality bias. A shadow of doubt pervades my spirit, yet I am aware of the re-emergence of a manful cry. The darkness, shadow is associated with evil and negativity, perpetuating racism. Who controls the power, the narrative of the feminine voice? The emergence of the feminine, speak to the voice of reason. Women are powerful healers, the cry of the earth resonates; powerlessness, war, the environment. The earth is crying for the voice of reason and healing; the dark mother before me has been suppressed, culture to culture eliminated. Emerge from fear, resolute in faith, trust in the moment; do not fear being seen, a valuable presence. Lovingly hold the spirit of the earth, the feminine, the feminine will hold you. I run to the feminine, cry and rush, push to reach recognizable arms that yearn to heal a fragmented existence.

Laurie G.
Workout #4

Type of Exercise: Running
Length of Exercise: 45 minutes
Music: Alphaville, "Forever Young"
Kind of Emotional Pain: The Ancestors Anguish

I begin my run reluctantly, anxious, and ready to leave Canada to return to San Francisco. I feel out of touch today, unfamiliar people, this environment makes me uneasy. The sun has a difficult time penetrating my thoughts, my breath is labored, lungs hurt the entire time I ran because I am desperate to run fast. Leave the past behind, I want to run faster, and leave the past behind. Whose past? Mine, my ancestors, I am aware that I have more choices than my grandmother, my life is easier. She traveled from Sweden to America when she was 13 years old, forced to leave Sweden because her family could not feed her. She was the oldest, therefore had to leave her family and friends. I have the diary she recorded of her adventure, but have yet to have it translated. I try to find her fear in my body, my heart. I am afraid to connect the fear and sadness she must have experienced. I imagine that I am her. Why didn't I ask her more questions, why was my family so unquestioning? Silence keeps us from knowing and expressing our deepest thoughts and experiences. Perhaps my silence is a distant expression of her sadness.

During her first workout, Laurie realizes that in her adolescence her parents silenced her by being unsupportive and discouraging. She addresses this issue in a generalized way, without getting into the specifics of what her parents actually did to silence her. Making a general statement about the cause of your emotional pain is an excellent starting point in a journal. Hopefully, as Laurie continues her journey, she will explore her childhood memories in fuller detail. During her third workout, Laurie connects with her struggle to find a voice with that of her female ancestors whom she joins in overcoming oppression. Laurie asserts that the historical oppression of women accounts for her own inability to speak out: History becomes destiny. It's a destiny she would alter, but in her fourth workout, speech again yields to silence; the silence of generations. Laurie connects with the spirit of her grandmother and sees her present-day silence as an expression of her grandmother's distant fear and sadness.

Laurie states that the Body-Mind-Soul Solution has given her tools to deal with her emotional issues. She has discovered that she had not previously been quite in touch with the conflicts in- side herself. She says, "This is different from traditional ther- apy where you talk and talk. The exercise allows you to experi- ence the emotional pain differently from being sedentary. It is an experience that integrates the emotional parts of us with the intellectual. I did not feel separated from my pain. I felt I could reach it or run through it."

Rhonda G., who was introduced in chapter 4, is a twenty-six- year-old African-American woman who faced the effects racism had on her during her workouts.

Rhonda G.
Workout #1

Type of Exercise: Running
Length of Exercise: 50–60 minutes
Music: Radio mix (rap, R&B, light rock, neo soul)
Kind of Emotional Pain: The Ancestors Anguish

Music helps. The more up-tempo, the more strength, drive and connectedness. I try to find something bigger than myself. While running, it crosses my mind that there are not a lot of people like me (Black Sistahs) running but rather Caucasians of all ages. What's up with that? Could it be a result of past/present geno- cide? It's sad! Why do I value exercise? I think that there is nihil- ism in my community, a kind of hopelessness carried over from extreme oppression and crushed dreams. But my mind shifts to resiliency and the matriarchs in my family and all the she-roes that defy psychological slavery and have paved the way for me. Because my ancestors were slaves and many of us suffer from psychological slavery, I GET MAD! I'm so tired of being the "only one" in a job setting, 7 out of 900 in a school setting—forced tokenism. I'm proud of my ancestry; luckily, I learned to love myself at an early age. Only God knows how different my life would be if I didn't.

Rhonda G.
Workout #2

Type of Exercise: Running
Length of Exercise: 50–60 minutes
Music: Radio mix (rap, R&B, light rock, neo soul)
Kind of Emotional Pain: The Ancestors Anguish

Running helped a lot today. I was pissed- –I'm the only person of color at my job and sometimes my co-workers make very offensive comments based on their ignorance. Running helps me shake off all that poison, sweat it out. During my run, I thought about relationships, specifically the difficulty black men and women have communicating. I'm sure some of my co-workers would think I'm being "hypersensitive," but in my mind there's a correlation between slavery and the emotional disconnect I encounter with some members of my own community. Today I passed a black man walking arm in arm with a white woman. I don't care who you date or who is your mate but, damn, last time I checked neither one of us is getting the respect we deserve. Hmm. While running, I recalled a statement a co-worker made. She said, "I don't understand the assumption that it is all about race." While running, I answered her. I was running fast, but I still answered her in my mind. "Of course you don't understand, how could you? You don't even acknowledge color. You said it yourself. 'I'm the norm.' You represent the dominant culture; everything outside that paradigm is OTHER. Don't tell me that I'm hypersensitive until you experience a day in my life."

After the mental chitchat, I slow my tempo and wonder how I am going to survive this world knowing what I know and being who I am. I smile. I know it will be a challenge but I have mountains to move. Tina Turner's song, "Simply the Best," hits the radio. I pick up the tempo and smoothly pass everyone that I can, making it look effortless. Thoughts of Ralph Ellison's *Invisible Man* cross my mind. Do these people even see me?

Rhonda G.
Workout #3

Type of Exercise: Walking
Length of Workout: 50–60 minutes
Music: Radio mix (rap, R&B, light rock, neo soul)
Kind of Emotional Pain: The Ancestors Anguish

Walking home from work always feels good. Leaving behind the poison and walking proud. A co-worker told me that I walk so proud like I don't take no mess. I imagine the ancestors walked this way. For once I agree with my co-workers. I do walk like I'm not going to be intimidated by anyone. Even better, my walk is filled with rhythm. Everything is about race for me and not because I choose it. The economic divide, joblessness, and ridiculously high incarceration rates are all connected to the genocide my people experienced. It is difficult, but the United States doesn't want, desire, or care to acknowledge slavery as genocide. In the National Holocaust Museum and in the Los Angeles Museum of Tolerance there is no acknowledgement of slavery. These things cross my mind, but I feel pumped. Alicia Keys is singing her new single. It's all good for now.

Rhonda G.
Workout #4

Type of Exercise: Walking
Length of Exercise: 50–60 minutes
Music: Radio mix (rap, R&B, light rock, neo soul)
Kind of Emotional Pain: The Ancestors Anguish

My car is broke down. Dealing with the "system" to get it fixed brings on stress. I try to let the music soothe my anxiety. I think about all those who came before me and how they stood up for their rights. I have a "plan of action" operation to get what I deserve!! I wonder will I always go through such mental exhaustion. Yep!! It's my plight, my people's plight. Did the ancestors believe in the United States? I know those who arrived here first didn't. Later generations didn't either, even once we were considered legitimate human beings. It seems that we have tried to make America work for us, but America refuses. What is the answer to this problem? Music—music straight don't mess with me posture. I am a token black with a little bit of access. I think back to Olympic hero Jesse Owens, Cuban sprinter Anna Quirot, and famed jurist Constance Baker Motley and walk on. The ancestors hold on to me and I hold on to them.

Music is an important element in Rhonda's healing process. It gives her strength, drive, and connectedness. It helps her work through the prejudice she deals with day-to-day, which she elaborates in her journal. She notes there, too, that she looks to her ancestors for strength and inspiration, and while she often walks (or runs) tough and proud, she nonetheless feels that she is invisible. Bringing imagination into therapeutic play, she scripts a make-believe dialogue between herself and an insensitive co-worker. This imaginary conversation enables her to release some of her bottled-up rage she has at her co-worker's attitude.

Rhonda finds the Body-Mind-Soul Solution to be liberating. "Asking myself questions while exercising was a positive thing that forced me to focus on my issues. Generally, I was thinking about the ancestors as synonymous with experiencing racism on a day-to-day basis. This program affirmed that I am coming to terms and have an increased awareness of the problems I am faced with. It has helped me realize that I need to discover nondestructive means for dealing with the inner pain around racism. I realized that dealing with racism will always be part of my life and utilizing the Body-Mind-Soul Solution is a healthy means to process it."

Sarah W., who we met in chapter 4, is a 43-year-old woman who uses the Body-Mind-Soul Solution to understand the origins of her low self-esteem and sense of powerlessness.

Sarah W.
Workout #1

Type of Exercise: Walking

Length of Exercise: 45 minutes

Emotional Pain Question: Why do I feel so powerless and why am I only seeing the negative?

For some reason, the day-to-day events of living are becoming very difficult and I feel stuck and unable to cope. I wonder how other people get through their day successfully without getting depressed. My therapist said that we can all choose how to deal with the stress. I know this, but have lost the concept along the way. I guess I slipped back to my old thinking of wanting to have everything lined up perfectly; neat, tidy, completed so I wouldn't have to worry about making mistakes or wrong decisions. I want to uncomplicate my life and thinking. I want to simplify and solve problems as they arise rather than seeing a problem as though I've made another mistake in judgment. That feeling is the familiar feeling I had growing up and even when I was still married to Randy. Why try to make things better when the end result is always the same—that you are a lousy piece of garbage, just taking up space.

Type of Exercise: Walking

Length of Exercise: 45 minutes

Emotional Pain Questions: Have I lost my young adult sons? Can I be satisfied with how I parented them? Why do I think that I am not finished with my job as a mother?

My dream last night left me with a feeling of helplessness. The very same physical and emotional feeling I had when I was being sexually abused. In my dream, I learned that my two sons had been abducted and were being sexually abused. When I finally got to them to help them, it was too late for my oldest boy, Tom. He didn't want to come back with me—he didn't want my help. He wanted to stay where he was. In fact, he wasn't really being sexually abused, but he was struggling and he wanted me to leave him there so he could struggle on his own without me. I was able to bring my younger son, Louis, back home with me, but it felt like he was also struggling with wanting to be with Tom. I wonder if that's what he feels in real life—like he has to connect with either me or Tom rather than break away and be on his own. Ironically, in my dream, I had asked my former husband to help me find the boys and bring them home. He said that he wanted to but couldn't because he had a 4 p.m. dentist appointment!

While walking, I was thinking that I need to look at my sons differently than as my little boys. If they were someone else's sons, I would regard them as adults. Additionally, I wouldn't look at Tom as a lost cause. I would see him as a rather nice guy who had some tough times growing up and is reacting normally. I wouldn't assume that his parents were failures because he does exhibit some positive and mature traits such as kindness and compassion. I want to stop feeling like I'm not done mothering. I want to stop feeling like I can find just the right words to say to Tom—he will see the light, go to college, have a successful career, strong relationship with a woman, and have a happy life. Like in my dream, I need to let him have his own struggles so he can learn life's lessons on his own. It's not black/white or pass/fail. I haven't lost him, but he is no longer open to my hand-holding and coddling. He wants to make it on his own. Watching Tom struggle is a helpless feeling for me, but I don't want to equate his helplessness with terror, dread, shame, embarrassment, and failure.

Sarah W.
Workout #3

Type of Exercise: Walking

Length of Exercise: 45 minutes

Emotional Pain Questions: Why do I feel so lonely? Why can't I reach out to someone to help ease the loneliness?

It's obvious to me that I've been using alcohol to deaden the pain of loneliness. Drinking emboldens me and takes away the fear of being alone. I was thinking that I still need to work on feeling and accepting the loss of my children, that that was the cause of my pain and loneliness. However, I know that my kids are behaving age-appropriate and I should and do feel proud of them as well as some pride for myself in how I raised them. After all, I spent 20 years of my life with and for them. They were my purpose in life. But, now I can see that it's not Tom and Louis I'm missing in my life—it's having a meaningful and enjoyable purpose in my life. I need to clarify within myself that I'm not lonesome. I have many friends who love me and want to spend time with me. Even my sons love me and occasionally want to spend time with me.

I guess I don't reach out to people because it's not really loneliness that I feel and when I think of contacting a friend, I think, "What's the use? It won't make me feel better." Plus, this negative attitude is very destructive to my mental health. I would like to look at my single lifestyle as opportunity and freedom to accomplish what I want to accomplish. A future with purpose—not just a future with a person. Whether it's having the time to learn how to make a soufflé, or volunteer in a school classroom, or design sewing patterns, it's my choice and my purpose, and it is all worthwhile. Looking at my life more positively doesn't feel so painful. And, less emotional pain makes drinking less desirable.

I've spent too many years looking for the right person to love and care for and give me a purpose.

It's 7:30 p.m. and I'm done writing this. Next, I'll return phone calls to my friends.

Type of Exercise: Walking
Length of Exercise: 45 minutes
Emotional Pain Questions: How did my family's poverty
                          and belief system affect me?

Hindu Caste System: the only way out of one's position is through death and reincarnation.

According to my parents and grandparents, I was born into a family whose station in life is just above the darkies and Indians. This was not a racial prejudice based on hatred or a sense of superiority, but rather a class issue. I felt comfort in my own class until I began to see a different world through my own eyes. Although my parents could interact with the people in the classes above us, they did so with respect and reverence—sort of like a child talking to an authority figure. Dad talking on the phone to his boss with a clear voice and no stuttering (my father was a stutterer all his life): "Yes, sir, Mr. Conyers. Thank you very much, Mr. Conyers." He would respond to the white collar (he considered himself blue collar) people at church: "Yes, Bob. I'd be happy to, Bob. I can do that for you, Bob. Thank you very much, Bob." He never spoke to his mom, his family, or his kids that way. With his kids it was, "Goddamn it, stop crying or I'll give you something to cry about. I don't care what you think; what I say goes, I'm going to put you over my knee."

Other people were treated respectfully; family didn't get any. My real world is the class which I was born into—a class not worthy of respect or privilege. Only others get that. I can only feel comfortable with nothing. That's where I belong.

I disassociate while I'm living in my privileged lifestyle. In my family's world, you are where you came from. Moving into another class is like changing one's height—it can't be done except by temporary, artificial means.

What is all this class crap? Who really cares?

This issue is not about whether or not I deserve to have material things, success, happiness, or fulfillment. The issue is being less than zero, being of negative value.

My inner core tells me that even if I won a million-dollar lottery and chose to give 99% of it away to my family and causes, it wouldn't change the way I perceive myself. I fear that I will always think of myself as silent, of no consequence, little value, a nuisance, and taking up space.

Sarah W.
Workout #5

Type of Exercise: Walking
Length of Exercise: 30 minutes
Emotional Pain Questions: I'm not even worth a five
minute conversation?

So, he hurt me again and he doesn't even know it; or does he? When I called yesterday, Dad never came to the phone to speak with me. Is this all a game with him? I don't ask for deep conversation or in-depth emotional interaction. I just want him to react to the cabin photos I sent two weeks ago. He has been a builder for over 60 years, so I thought he'd enjoy seeing the construction progress of my new home. He doesn't give and he doesn't take. His silence kills.

I've been unsuccessfully trying to please my father for 55 years. This is the first man of any importance to me. He was supposed to be my teacher and my protector but it didn't happen that way. I feel like a kicked dog. And just like a dog that offers unconditional love to its owner, I forget about the last injury and return with only the intent of pleasing. With unrealistic expectations and young-girl-like fantasy, I've been trying to maintain this totally skewed father-daughter relationship which has caused me years of pain and self-doubt.

So how do I ease the pain? Is this really pain?

My father is a big screw-up and I've come pretty far in life totally on my own and without him. Why do I let his frozen alcoholic heart impact me now? I guess I'm not feeling actual pain; more like an internal ache, perhaps a feeling of grief for the loss of a very worn and tired-out fantasy. As with my mother, I must have no expectations of my father. The occasional bone he throws my way is merely accidental or only to foster his own sense of self-worth. The problem is with my father, not with me. To continue seeking love and acceptance from my father is futile and self-destructive.

Type of Exercise: Walking

Length of Exercise: 45 minutes

Emotional Pain Questions: Why am I angry at my father?

My angry feelings toward my father are mixed and stirred up with my angry feelings toward my ex-husband. I was conditioned to accept neglect and condescension as a way of life because I am female; it is my duty/responsibility to ensure that my father, brothers, grandfather, uncles, male cousins, priests, male friends are treated with respect and gratitude and superior reverence—somewhat like a master-slave relationship.

On a conscious level, I know this is inaccurate. However, on a deeper level, I feel that an enormous rage is now surfacing because of this "training." A better word might be brainwashing. I feel like a prisoner with both fists clutching at the prison bars, screaming to be let free. I feel like I have been falsely imprisoned—whatever crime I am accused of, I DIDN'T DO IT! I'm innocent and need to be set free. I need to live life as a free person, as a free human being without the shackles of gender inequality. I don't want to be devalued because I supposedly lack physical strength or am deemed to have inferior intelligence because I'm a girl.

I have proven myself over and over again. I am physically and emotionally strong. I'm intelligent, empathetic, and environmentally conscious. Give me a freakin' break! Neither my father nor my ex nor any of my brothers are that way. Also, I'm emotional, compassionate, spiritual, loving, and maternal. I want to embrace these traits, yet doing so makes me feel weak. In other words, being female makes me feel weak and inferior. How do I balance this dichotomy?

Sarah W.
Workout #7

Type of Exercise: Walking

Length of Exercise: 45 minutes

Emotional Pain Questions: Why did I make it my job to protect my father from his own suffering?

It is difficult for me to get to the place where I held his pain, his suffering, and his depression. It hurts me to know that I had to forfeit my childhood so he wouldn't feel his own childhood pain. How unfair that I felt it my lot to protect him from his suffering. Expressing an opinion or view that might conflict with his was taboo because it might upset him, thus boomerang the pain back to me.

He didn't reconcile with his own demons: his poverty-stricken upbringing, his alcoholic father and co-dependent mother, his lack of education and societal mores, his speech impediment, his emotional depression, his own alcoholism. These were the traits my father exhibited and for some reason I felt compelled to protect him from the pain of these realities. He was never my protector, but more like a benefactor. One to whom I needed to show gratitude and admiration, as if I were a foster child and taking on his pain was the only way I could repay him for allowing me to live in my home. I had no other means of compensation for my existence. I can't continue paying down the debt. Being born was not my idea, nor was it my fault. I want to be emotionally debt-free from my mother and father.

How this warped sense of duty to others has manifested itself throughout my adult life is pretty clear. Time to work on it!!!

The seven entries in Sarah's journal examine the origins of her emotional pain. Notice how each entry becomes a prerequisite for the next and how she addresses her emotional pain immediately throughout each time she writes. It is apparent from the onset that Sarah realizes she has always experienced low self-esteem. She feels that she is not even worthy of human consideration; that she is "a lousy piece of garbage." During the second workout, she painfully examines her relationship with her two sons with some ambivalence and acknowledges that her responsibility for them has diminished since they've become young adults. If in her second journal entry she identifies herself in terms of her two sons, as a mother, in the third, she begins to define her identity as an independent self. No longer is her primary function to be a caretaker; nor does she want it to be. Nor does she want her current course to be obfuscated, as it sometimes is, by loneliness and alcohol, neither of which can heal nor resolve her emotional pain. During the fourth workout, Sarah delves into extraordinary painful, for her, subject of class, more particularly the lower working class into which she was born and which emotionally she has never left, despite her now "privileged lifestyle." Her economic and social accomplishments do not impress her father in any case, and in her fifth workout she has to come to terms with his emotional abandonment, which has been devastating to her. She mourns the lack of an emotionally present father, but she also now recognizes that the dynamic of her trying to get him to notice her has been totally destructive. She vows she'll stop seeking his love and acceptance. In the sixth journal entry, Sarah broadened her perspective on her problem by viewing low self-esteem as a woman's problem; for by their fathers, husbands, bosses, priests, politicians, men have made women to feel like second-class citizens. Venting her anger, she determines to stop internalizing this inferior image of females. During her seventh workout, Sarah explores further her relationship with her father as she focuses on her lifelong attempts to protect him from his own suffering. What she saw as her duty was in fact her only way of connecting with her emotionally distant father, and the only way she could "protect" him was to take on his anguish as her own. She decides that protection is no longer her responsibility and that it is an impossible task, and in the resolve she begins to set herself free.

Sarah feels that the Body-Mind-Soul Solution has been instrumental to her healing. It enabled her not only to separate herself emotionally from her dysfunctional parents, but also at the same time she was able to establish healthy boundaries with her sons. For years Sarah had been diagnosed with major depression and anxiety. She was taking large doses of antidepressant medication. She was drinking to excess. The Body-Mind-Soul Solution provided her a tool that helped to get free of these dependencies and at the same time heal her emotional pain.

Alice W., who was introduced in chapter 4, is a twenty-nine-year-old woman who is grieving the death of her father.

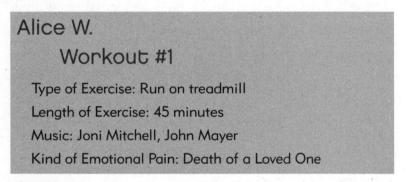

Alice W.
Workout #1
Type of Exercise: Run on treadmill
Length of Exercise: 45 minutes
Music: Joni Mitchell, John Mayer
Kind of Emotional Pain: Death of a Loved One

I'm exercising at a fitness facility in a hotel during a work-related trip. I am thinking of my father because of all the time he spent in hotels. The Joni Mitchell songs remind me of him because he loved her music. I feel emotional. I wish I could call him to talk about my trip, about my career, about business travel. He traveled A LOT! His sudden death by heart attack was so painful because I never got to ask him so many things. I think I would have been able to ask, had I known I only had limited time. I think so

much about "growing up" and how it feels to have more responsibilities, more plans to make. Big decisions. How did he know
whether to get married or have kids?

Alice W.
Workout #2

Type of Exercise: Run 3–4 miles

Length of Exercise: 45 minutes

Music: Hip hop, John Mayer

Kind of Emotional Pain: Death of a Loved One

We are running outside in Memphis. I am with my partner Sa-
mantha's family. Her dad is going to come to San Francisco to run
a marathon with her. I feel jealous that her dad can support her
and be able to be close to her in that way. I didn't get to live away
from home long enough when my dad was alive to develop a new
and more adult kind of relationship with him.

I miss telling him about highs and lows of work, friendships, and
relationships. I need his advice and guidance. I can't find anyone
who is as smart and as grounded. I can't find anyone who I trust to
be as encouraging and knowledgeable in the way that he was.

The dance music and the heat/humidity make for a very intense exercise experience.

Alice W.
Workout #4

Type of Exercise: Run on a treadmill
Length of Exercise: 30 minutes
Music: Dance Music
Kind of Emotional Pain: Death of a Loved One

It is my birthday today. I spoke to my mom on the phone before my workout. She announced that she is planning to sell our home. It's time, actually. She has far too much space and the house probably is preventing her from "moving forward." She does have a new boyfriend. I want to think of a reason to be angry at her—to tell her she is being selfish. I feel lonely. I know my sister will be upset. She lives near my mom and spends a lot of time at the house. What is happening to my family? My mom in an apartment; a new stepdad, maybe? Also, how will she manage this huge undertaking of selling a home and moving away all by herself? Shall I offer to come home and help her pack? Shall I help her with her financial plans? I am running hard and fast and I cry a bit when I get to the locker room.

In working out, Alice is working through the emotionally painful loss of her father. She regrets not having made the time to discuss important issues with her dad. She misses his wisdom, guidance, love, kindness, and she really misses them intensely more when she observes the relationship her partner shares with her father.

Alice has been deeply wounded by the abruptness of her father's death by heart attack, but she now is able to process the notion that although he is deceased, she can give herself permission to experience joy. Yet she does not give in easily, to herself or to her mother, who is attempting to move on. Still, Alice knows that moving on is a normal process and with the Body-Mind-Soul Solution she too is beginning to move forward.

Alice says, "Exercise takes me to a place where I trust myself. I recorded my thoughts in my journal after I was done working out. The writing part helped even though it was difficult to sit down. I was happy and proud that I could write it down and put my thoughts out into the world. The Body-Mind-Soul Solution gave me the space to reflect on what I went through after his death and how difficult it was and therefore I am not so hard on myself."

Bob Livingstone

Type of workout: Running
Length of Exercise: 40 minutes
Music: Beggars Banquet — The Rolling Stones
Kind of Emotional Pain: Stuck Grief
Emotional Pain Question: Today is my birthday and why
do I feel so bad?

Happy Birthday to Us

Today is my birthday.

I don't feel like celebrating.

People wish me well, but I'm not feeling it.

I'm not the man I want to be and teach others to become.

I don't live in the moment and am often racked with all-consuming fear;

The anxiety of what is going to happen next sometimes kills me.

I don't feel like I deserve to celebrate the day of my birth.

I want to disappear when people smile at me.

I don't know what's wrong.

I should be very happy.

I'm in love,

I'm in great health,

But something is holding me back.

I'm listening to "Salt of the Earth" by the Stones.

I have a memory of my father entering the front door of my house.

Why was he coming home from work so early?

He had his gray work shirt, khakis, and black boots on,

His hair was flying all over his head underneath a white cotton cap,

He had a dazed look in his eyes that no one would talk about.

Later my mother told me that my dad got fired from his job because he forgot to tell them he was going on vacation:

Something was wrong with his brain.

Something the doctor knew about but would not fix.

My father, swatted away from his factory job,

Like a fly meeting the swatter;

My father, neglected by the health care system and finally, callously thrown into a hole dug in the New Jersey earth for departure unknown;

My father, men, and women like him who created the goods that made our life so much easier.

My father was treated like a replaceable part in the factory, discarded when no longer useful.

His final days were not filled with grace,

His funeral was undignified and hateful,

His dreams would never be uttered from his lips again;

All that was left was disappointment, hurt, and shame.

It has been my quest to erase this shame from the eternal past.

I want my father's life and all those who have been disregarded to have faces, to have names, to be visible and strong;

I want to go back and ease my father's burden, to make him happy and proud of who he was and where he came from;

I want him to shed his fears and agony;

I want him to know he was loved,

Not only by me, my mother, and sister,

But appreciated by the whole world.

"Salt of the Earth" both mocks and honors the working class;

My mood dictates which aspect I pay attention to.

I can't bring honor to my father by my own success as a therapist, a writer, a man;

I cannot change the horrid past no matter what I do.

I should know this by now, but it doesn't surprise me that I have not accepted what happened.

How can I honor my own worth, my own achievement, if my father died without experiencing his real value?

Do I have the right to enjoy the riches that this life holds if my father did not get the opportunity?

I hit the streets running hard. It has been raining all week and this is the first day in a while the sun has shown its face.

The new Al Green is on the iPod and the title track, "It's OK," is pouring into my ears like hot lava.

I look up at the bright sky while the fullness of soul music fills my heart. The heavens part and the voice of my father rings out. He says, "It has been a long time since we talked, son. It has been so gallant of you to fight my fight for me, but I want to tell you that my life was not tragic. I did discover a love so strong. Few men have been fortunate to have the love I shared with your mother. I also loved you and your sister. You see, son, family was all that was important to me.

"You can rest now. You can be at peace. You can continue to fight the fight, but you don't have to do it for me any more. The way I lost my job, how I was slowly losing my mind, and how dispiriting my funeral was does not matter now. I want you to know that I did attain dignity in my life, the highest form of dignity one can have—the ability to love unconditionally and the willingness to let others love me. All that matters and what I want to pass on to you is the willingness to allow this joy to fill your life.

"So celebrate life, celebrate your life, but you don't have to do it for me. I know you miss me, especially when something exciting happens or when you feel lost. You will always miss me, as I you."

I see my father sitting in a white wicker chair. He is wearing white linen pants, sandals, and a Kweejiboe blue and green shirt. He has a serene look on his face. The tropical breeze gives him relief from the heat. He is in paradise, someplace like the Gulf of Mexico. He is drinking a Ramos fizz. He raises his glass to toast.

"Let's drink to the hard-working millions. Let's drink to the salt of the earth. Happy Birthday, Rob."

Before I began this workout, I was feeling numb, restless, out of sorts, and nothing about this special day, my fifty-fifth birthday, made me the least bit happy. Everyone and everything were managing to get on my nerves. I was agitated, short of temper. My verbal responses were curt and I felt like my brain was underwater. I hated feeling this way and wanted to do something to alter my dismal mood.

So I forced myself to get off the couch and into my running gear with my latest MP3 player. Before I headed out to the streets for my five-mile run, I had no hope that I would find any answers or solace. I usually begin my run at a relatively fast pace for an almost senior citizen (I can buy groceries at a discount in some locations at age fifty-five). On this day, too, I ran hard and immediately surrendered to my distress. Again the memories of my father's last days on earth visited me; memories held deep in my mind and heart. Again I was so saddened by the undignified manner in which he was fired from his job and by the humiliating experience that his funeral was. Again I was driven by my need to redeem the last final days of my dad's life. I had to prove that his firing was unjust and I had to get him a better job. I had to somehow undo his empty and insulting funeral. I ran, but I was being driven.

Up to this point in my life, I had been unaware that in all my efforts to be successful I was trying somehow to redeem my father. I now faced for the first time the realization that this drive had disguised itself as the dreadful anxiety that I experienced every day when I awoke. It was a feeling that always defied words. Now I had the words, and I realized that I couldn't save him, ever. He was dead. Yet I could talk to his spirit. And did.

That birthday journey included a soundtrack. It was the Rolling Stones' *Beggars Banquet*. It played as my tears fell and my father gently told me to let him go.

Chapter Nine

Conclusion: How to Make the Body-Mind-Soul Solution an Essential Part of Your Life

I have been practicing techniques from the Body-Mind-Soul Solution since 2002, nearly four years now. The Body-Mind-Soul Solution has become an essential part of my life because I have learned and continue to learn valuable lessons about healing from it. They have altered my everyday life in vital, constructive ways:

- When I feel emotionally numb, I no longer allow myself to remain so for a minute's worth of time. Indeed, the moment I realize that I am "emotionally constipated," I immediately begin to utilize the program. In this situation I start with the emotional pain question, "Why am I having difficulty feeling anything?" In the course of my run, I unfailingly come up with the answer.

- I have become much more self-aware. I am now more in touch with my thoughts and my feelings, so that I can mindfully respond to whatever is stirring up confusion and angst inside me. Being self-aware is the first step in resolving problems. It is also key in dealing with anger directed toward another. If you are self-aware, you will recognize that the first feeling to strike you in the rage cycle is hurt. Awareness of that fact enables you to understand more readily why you are hurt and to address the cause in an appropriate manner with others.

- I now have many fewer illnesses related to stress. I used to frequently suffer sinus headaches and various muscle pains because I was holding on to fear. Since I have discovered a means through The Body-Mind-Soul Solution to let the fear go, I am not continually plagued with stress-related physical pain.

- I have become a much more patient person. I am now able to take the time necessary to process ideas. I used to be so fear-based that I would skip blindly over essential steps that could have helped me and spared me much emotional pain along the way. I was also very impatient with others. I have learned to relax more frequently and experience joy more fully.

- I have continued to realize and expand the power of my voice of wisdom in that higher place within, the psyche, or soul. Most of my life I didn't believe in anything spiritual and I certainly was too cynical to believe in God. The realization of my spiritual dimension is a work in progress. I do believe firmly that energy greater than what we call human that runs through and outside of us. I am beginning to believe that if I can give up my instinct or need to control and surrender to this energy, it will lead me to my true self-loving center. While I am not there yet, I am ready to take whatever the next step may be.

Allow the Body-Mind-Soul Solution to play an essential role in your life. Whenever you are sedentary and suddenly faced with a perplexing problem, recall the calm, brave state you have reached through exercise. Remember how confident you felt while exercising and remember, too, the sweat streaming from your pores and the tears that streamed with it. Recall your workouts when all the different facets of your being were performing in harmony and confusion had been banished. Remember the new insights you discovered and the plans you formulated to deal with your emotional pain. Review your journals, track your emotional transformation and appreciate the lessons you have learned.

The Body-Mind-Soul Solution can help you transform self-doubt to hope. It can give you the strength of the following convictions as you go through each day:

- You have the right to have a successful and peaceful life.

- You have the ability to identify, face, and work through your emotional pain.

- You now know that pushing away emotional pain is ultimately more harmful than dealing with it.

- You now realize that you are the only person that can heal yourself, but instead of viewing that insight with despair, you embrace it.

You can make the Body-Mind-Soul Solution an integral part of your daily life by implementing it whenever you feel out of sorts but don't know exactly why; when unresolved childhood issues arise; distressing personal tragedies and relationship break-ups occur, or when the anniversary dates of major losses arrive.

You now have the tools to bring joy into your life.

The Body-Mind-Soul Solution: Healing Emotional Pain through Exercise

JOURNAL ENTRY FORM

Name:

Workout #:

Date:

Type of Exercise:

Length of Exercise:

Music Selection:

Issue (please circle one) Stuck Grief, Death of a Loved One, The Teenager Within, Anger that Hurts Those You Love, The Ancestors Anguish, other _____

Emotional Pain Question:

Journal notes after workout:

[You can print copies of this form by going to www.boblivingstone.com]